Heal Yourself Holistically

Your Herb & Crystal Guide

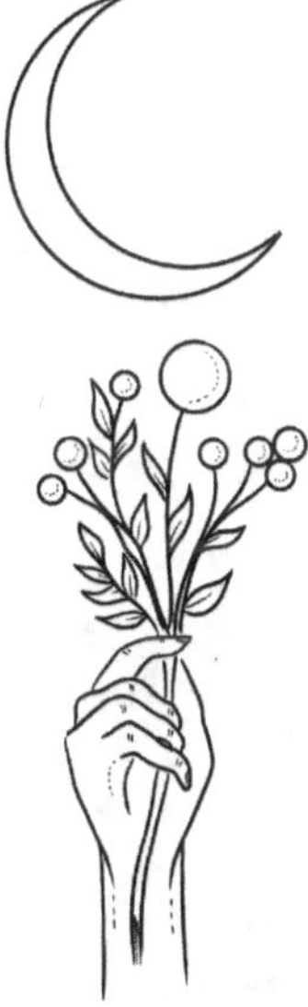

Bridget M. Shoup

Illustrations: Jared A. Shoup

Photography: Kelsey K. Shoup

ISBN: 9798651526574

~ "Heal Yourself Holistically" ~ Bridget M. Shoup ~

DEDICATION

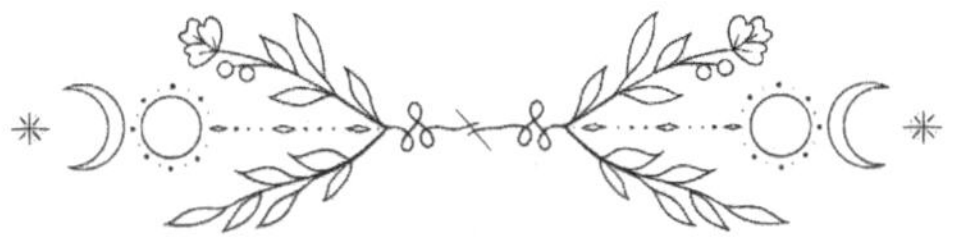

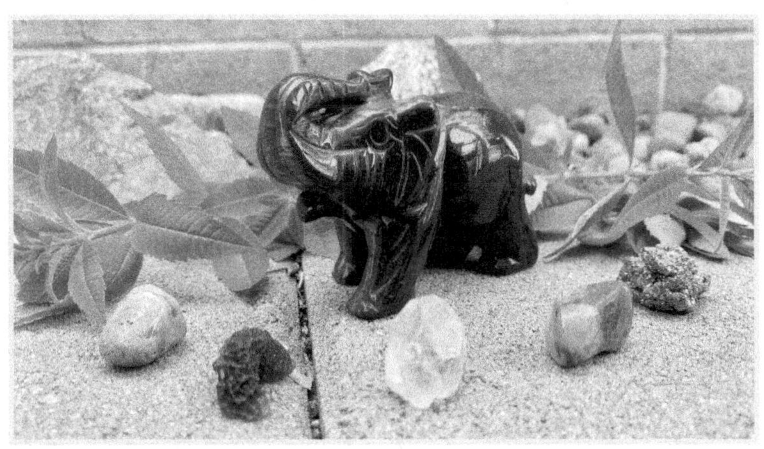

This book is Dedicated to My Loves,
Jared & Kelsey.
Love you both to the Moon & Back... Infinity & Beyond!

Also...
To the amazing Souls out there
seeking alternative methods to heal yourself & your loved ones!

May this book help guide you in finding
happiness & healing!

CONTENTS

INTRODUCTION

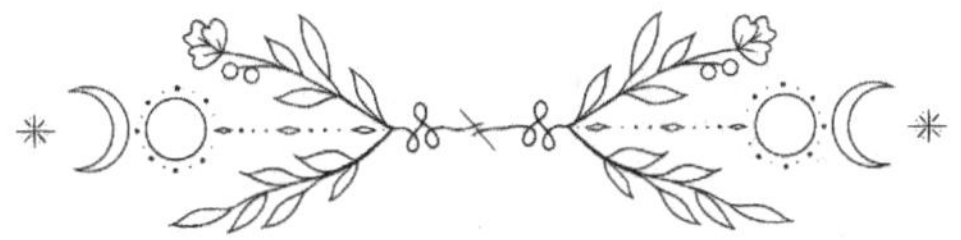

We are so blessed to have such an abundant Earth! The Mother to us all... Gaia!!

From the ground in which we find stability, to the plants and minerals that inhabit all corners of this planet!

Most people might take the weeds in their garden for granted, but did you know they actually have a purpose? A function to help us heal ourselves holistically!!

Weeds (Dandelions) can in fact heal us!!
From Menopausal symptoms to dissolving Kidney Stones & Gallbladder issues, Dandelions are here to resolve these issues and so many more!

Plants are here on the Earth's surface for our use and consumption. But Minerals, or more commonly known as Crystals... are deep within Gaia offering amazing healing benefits as well!

One of the most commonly found Crystal is Clear Quartz!
Clear Quartz are not only used in our computers, tablets and cell phones, but they also help our watches and clocks keep time too!

And did you know, Clear Quartz Crystals are even in the lighters for kitchen stoves! (that ticking sound you hear strikes against Quartz to help it light)

These are just some of the applications of Clear Quartz in our world today!

In addition to helping us with everyday life things, they are also very powerful as a healing tool!!

Known as the "Master Healer", Clear Quartz speeds up the healing process of any aliment that you might be faced with!

This book will help you discover all the fascinating ways that Herbs and Crystals are here to assist us heal our Minds, Bodies & Spirit!

Buckle up, and let's dive into the Magickal world of the Plant Kingdom & Mineral Kingdom… as we learn ways to "Heal Yourself Holistically!"

MY STORY

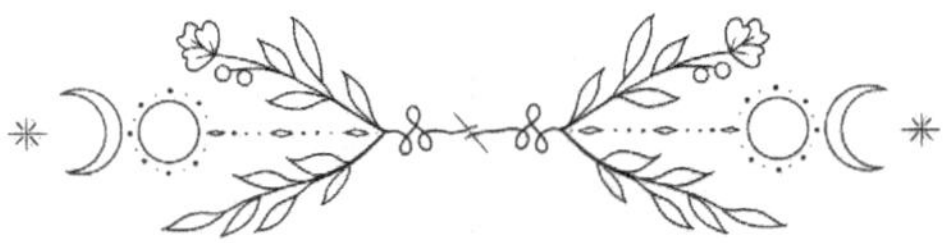

I have always been the type of Soul who would seek out alternative ways to heal myself and family! To this day, it's our main way of dealing with any medical challenges that we might be faced with!

As a kid growing up, my Mom introduced me to the world of herbs. Starting out with the more common type herbs like Lavender. She would make things that we would keep in our pillowcases or in our room to not only fill the room with a lovely fragrance, but to actually help relax us for sleep time.

Not realizing the benefits at the time, I didn't entertain learning more about herbs until later in life. Fast forward....

2013 was the beginning of my Spiritual Awakening! During that time, things started to change dramatically in my life, in positive ways of course. Little by little I was starting to see things differently, my eye (third eye) was beginning to open!!

I started working with Crystals and realized how powerful these little friends are! Transforming mine and my families life in astonishing ways!! Helping us heal!!
Believe me, my Hubby & Daughter got sick of hearing... "hey, there's a Crystal for that!" But it was true!!

I for one was so excited to see how much Crystals could heal us, that I wanted to scream it from the roof tops!! How the heck does no one talk about this? Do people know that Crystals can heal us, and with no side effects, well except for feeling better!?

From there, it was on!! I was on a mission to learn and educate myself with as much information as I could get my hands on!

I dove deep into learning as much as I could about Crystals. Enrolled in courses, became a Crystal Reiki Master… and to this day share my healing gifts with others. I travel to people's homes and offices to offer my services with my company called B*MoonStruck ! (www.BMoonStruck.com)

Down the rabbit hole I went, and soon after learning about Crystals… Herbs came into my radar. Remembering the seeds that were planted earlier in my childhood…working with Herbs came quite naturally for me!

Just like Crystals… Herbs also have powerful healing effects!
From creating potions (essential oil & crystal blends) that helped relieve sore muscles and pain, to crafting my own teas from the herbs I grow in my garden… I started to rely on Herbs just as much as my Crystal Friends!

Just as before, I started taking classes to learn more about Herbs and Essential oils. Being a Certified Aromatherapist & Herbalist now, working with Plant Medicine has become a big part of my healing practice!

From there, I also started to teach classes on Crystal healing to share my knowledge with others! After that, I was inspired by my Spirit Guides to write my first book called, "Crystal Clear Enlightenment" A Guide to Spiritual Growth. My mission is to assist as many people as I can live a happier, healthier holistic lifestyle. Writing my 1st book was another way to share with others.. near and far!

As time has carried on, again… I was feeling the nudge to write!
Could this be? Should I write a 2nd book now?? I just released my 1st book on 02/02/2020, is it too soon?

But, when Spirit speaks…I listen!
Off to writing book #2!! I feel so strongly to empower people with knowledge on how to heal themselves. In this way, you won't have to rely so heavily on others (Doctors, Pharmacies, etc). This is a way to take your power back and learn to heal yourself!

This book is a guide book to help you along your healing journey! I have always wanted a book that combined both Herbs and Crystals together, with their information on how they heal. Thus, my book "Heal Yourself Holistically" was born!

I'm wishing you and your family health and wellness always! May this book guide you in finding good health.

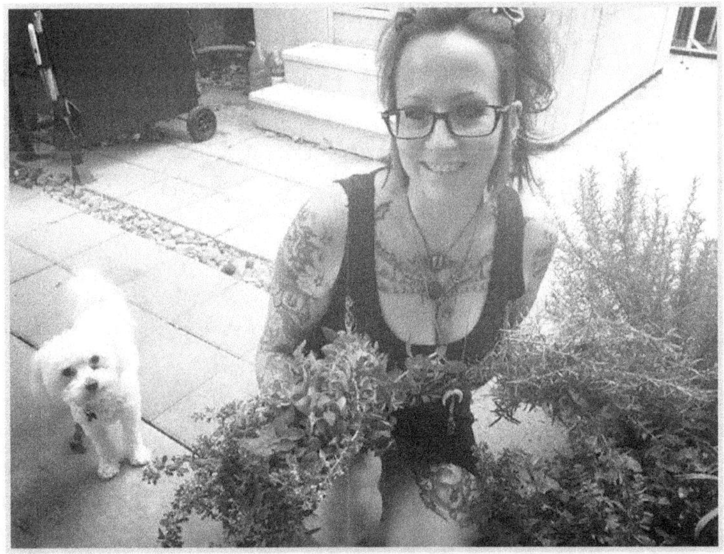

Let's Get Personal…

I want to share a few personal stories with you on how Crystals and Herbs have benefited mine and my families life!

Anxiety

In my personal life, I work with Crystals (quite a few I might add) everyday! I don't leave home without my sparkly little friends! Being an Empath, somedays it's hard for me to be out in groups of people. I rely on my Shungite and Lepidolite for days like that, but in addition to that… I layer on some Herbs!! My favorite Herb to work with to relax myself and releases any stress or anxiety is Ashwagandha. Not only is it helpful in those areas, but it also boosts the immune system and has anti-aging effects… oh and enhances your memory!! Win-Win-Win-Win!!!

Other things I do to help myself is I use my potion that I created…. called "Calm Diggy-Diggy".

It's an essential oil blend of Lavender, Frankincense and Amethyst Crystal. I just roll it on, take a few deep breaths in… and feel so much better!

You can order yours in my shop, Bridget's Brew.

(www.etsy.com/shop/bridgetsbrew)

Pain

Now for my Husband, he has had 3 (yes 3) knee surgeries! Of course when you have knee surgeries the Doctors always prescribe something to help you deal with the pain. He started norcos back in 2002 when he had his 1st knee surgery. Back then of course, I hadn't been "Enlightened" yet… so I had no idea we had all these amazing Herbal & Crystal options!

As I said, he had been on norcos (an opiate) since 2002. Every once in a while he felt like he needed to detox. Now let me tell you… if you have ever been around someone who is detoxing, it's most certainly NO fun!

The first few times he detoxed, he would do it cold turkey! Yikes right!?

It was no fun for him, or us!

As My hubby started to see the positive change in me as I continued to work with Crystals, he asked if I could help him get off his pills? I said, "of course!"

So in July 2016 we started the process.

First thing was first, I made him a Crystal Elixir (Water infused with Crystal energy) I worked with Amethyst to remove addiction and to add a sense of calm as he went through the detoxing process. I also added in a Clear Quartz Crystal to help him have clarity of mind, and to speed up the process.

He immediately started drinking the Crystal Elixir I had made for him. Now, the interesting thing was I knew he was drinking it, as I would refill it once he finished it. I did NOT know how he was doing with tapering down off the pills. Was he cutting back?? I didn't want to ask!

All I knew was that he was acting like he normally did. Not like before when he detoxed! After about a few weeks, I asked him how he was doing with cutting back on his pills? He said he cut back, but he's doing it little by little.

I didn't want to bug him too much, as he was going through this detoxing process!

Fast forward to Sept. 2016 and checking back in with him after 3 months time, he went from taking 6 norcos a day to only 2!! That was huge!! For him to reduce his pills that much and feeling great, that was a huge success right there!

But.. it gets better!!

Checking back in with him Oct. 2016, he was now only taking 1 pill a day. He still continued to drink his Crystal Elixir each day (sometimes multiple times a day, as he felt he needed it.)

But wait… there is more!

We had learned about an Herbal supplement called Kratom from his pain management Doctor. His Doctor knew we were more about the holistic approach to things.

My Hubby was all about it, "I'm going to give it a try! Maybe it will be what I need to get off these pills 100%!!" he said.

Oct. 2018 he started taking Kratom, and guess what? No more norcos! To this day (2020), he continues to work with Crystals, drinks Crystal Elixirs and takes herbal supplements to deal with any discomfort he might be experiencing.

No more going to the pain management Doctor .
(he literally quit going to him after that 1st month of taking Kratom)!!
No more paying the high price for the prescription pills!
No more Doctor visit bills!
No more feeling out of it, and yucky from his pills!

Kratom is a Herb that grows in Southeast Asia. It's related to the coffee bean and has stimulating qualities to it. It's known to boost your energy, helps you deal with anxiety and depression, as well as eliminates pain.

My Hubby reported feeling better than he ever had taking the norcos! I'm so happy for him! He honestly is healthier and happier than ever before!! I know we can thank the Crystals and Herbs for that!

Crohn's

Now onward to my Daughter's story!

When my Daughter was 8 years old (2008) she became quite sick. When we would go to the Doctor they would tell me she was "fine" according to their blood work (looking for viral & bacterial infections).

But something was defiantly NOT right! She was loosing weight, constantly going to the bathroom and would sleep most of the day away due to lack of energy.

I started to research her symptoms and found a diagnoses of Crohn's. I mentioned it to her Doctor, and her Doctor agreed we should have her looked at by a GI Doctor. (GI=Gastrointestinal)

At the age of 8, she was diagnosed with Crohn's disease!

I really had NO idea what the heck that was. Just the little bit of information that I had found online. How do we treat this? Will she be ok? All these thoughts start to enter my mind!

If you aren't familiar, Crohn's disease is an auto immune disease. Basically her immune system is fighting her intestines... as her immune system believes her intestinal tract to be foreign in her body. This causes ulcers within her intestinal tract, which in turn causes pain when digesting food, diarrhea, weight loss, pain in the abdomen, low energy, and constant trips to the restroom. Some people also experience bleeding from their anus as another sign.

This is said to be incurable, and treated with medications. The goal is to achieve remission, meaning her Crohn's isn't actively flaring. As when she is in remission, she has no ulcers inflamed that cause her problems.

They put her on some heavy steroids (prednisone) and something called Sulfasalazine, which would help with the inflammation in her intestines.

It did help her, and after weening off the steroids and staying on Sulfasalazine for 3 years, she was able to taper off of them… as she had achieve remission!

All was well until 2017, the year of her high school graduation.

You see, one of the triggers for a Crohn's flare up … is … Stress!!
Yep, she was stressing out about the whole "after high school" fears they like to feed our kids in school. I of course did my best to assure her, nothing was going to change… it would just be better, because she didn't HAVE to go to school! hahaha!

But again, you can only offer your loved ones the information.
They have to want to change, and sometimes change is hard!
She was open and willing to work with Crystals and we started right away!

As the previous symptoms started to creep in, I was well versed in Crystal healing at this point… so we got right to helping her with Crystals in a variety of ways!

I would do Crystal Chakra Balancing sessions with her, made her a Crystal Elixir with Blue Chalcedony (known to help relax and heal the intestines) as well as made a Crystal Grid for her healing. She started to actively work with Crystals at this time! The Crystal I knew would help her the most was Chrysocolla. This beauty is known to help heal the intestines as well as relive any stomach/intestinal cramping.

It started to make a huge difference for her!
However, the stress overcame her and she ended up in the hospital for 1 week a few days after graduation!

It was a tuff time of course, but we where grateful she was able to walk and graduate with her friends! We are also grateful that she got to learn from this experience, as she was too young to recall how it felt before this time.

During the hospital stay they where trying to push one of the highest, harshest drugs that helps treat Crohn's… Remicade!

Now, if you have ever seen the tv commercials on this drug... it's known to cause cancer! Ummmm, no thanks!

We denied and opted for Sulfasalazine again.
After she was released she continued on the pills till about 2018.

The pills where starting to really bother her stomach. So we started looking into alternative Herbal supplements she could take instead, along with working with her Crystals.

After much research, I came up with some Herbal options.

First we started with Boswellia and Turmeric, both excellent in removing inflammation within the body! She also started taking Slippery Elm.
Slippery Elm is great, it releases a gel-like substance that will line the intestines. It's beneficial if you have ulcers or Crohn's/Colitis because it gives your body a break and allows the food to pass through without aggravation.
She was making progress, but needed more!

Onward to Wormwood!
Wormwood is great for people with IBD/IBS as it helps treat the issues that comes along with the disease. In fact, it's equivalent to taking Remicade/Humaria (prescription drugs usually prescribed for people with IBD).
Wormwood has also been studied to be more effective than steroids!

The thing about Wormwood though, is you have to be very careful with it!It's NOT meant for long term use! You should only take it for 1 month as recommended, and then take 1 month break off of it!
Failure to do so can result in very less than desired side effects!
Just don't roll that dice!

However, when she started to take the Wormwood....she noticed immediate results! It made a huge difference!

Since you can only take Wormwood every other month or so, it was important to find other herbal supplements she could take when she wasn't taking Wormwood.

That led us to the following:
The * items she takes daily!

- *Marshmallow Root (helps with digestive upset & is an anti-inflammatory)
- Milk Thistle (when needed for stomach upset & aids in intestinal discomfort)
- Ginger Root (Great for inflammation, Indigestions & stomach upset)
- *L-Glutamine (Calms joint discomfort, helps digestive tract)
- Wormwood (treats IBD symptoms)
- *Turmeric (anti-inflammatory)
- *Boswellia (anti-inflammatory & helps with cramping)
- Evening Primrose (helps with cramping esp. when period near/on)
- Bentonite Clay (intestinal issues, helps w/diarrhea)
- Slippery Elm (coats intestines and relaxes stomach)
- *Multi Vitamin
- *Vitamin B12
- *Vitamin D
- *Vitamin C
- *Fish Oil
- Intestinal Comfort Tea (Herbal Mixture of: Dandelion Leaf, St. John's Wort, Lemon Balm Leaf, Calendula Flowers, Fennel Seed)
- *CBD Oil (relaxation for bed time/pain reliever)
- Gaba (as needed for anxiety & to relieve stress)
- *Qing Dai (heals intestines, mucosal healing)

Now I should note, she doesn't take ALL of these daily... but almost! Some days if her stomach feels fine she won't take say.. the Ginger or Milk Thistle.

As you see, I *stared the things she takes daily.
The un-starred Herbs she takes as needed.

And once every other month is on Wormwood in addition to the other Herbs/vitamins.

It might seem like quite a long list but, it has made a huge difference in how she feels. Her pain has subsided and she has more energy with less joint pains and Crohn's symptoms. It's worth it!

As you learn this information you will probably feel like me and want to share it was everyone you know. There is nothing wrong with that, just don't get down on yourself if someone isn't quite ready to take that next step in healing themselves holistically. It's not your responsibility. That is up to them. Sometimes all it takes is planting that seed of knowledge, and when the time is right that person will come back to it!

They have to be ready and willing with an open mind to want to heal themselves.
Once they are ready, amazing transformation can happen!

There is nothing wrong with continuing to use western medicine as well, but it's good to know there are so many alternative options out there for you! In fact, working with both herbs and crystals in conjunction with western medicine fit together well.

As you have read, my family turns to the assistance of herbs and crystals as our goto for healing!

Mind blowing results… time and time again from the assistance of Herbs and Crystals…. have lead me to create this book for you!

I wanted to write a book that would combine the two worlds, Plant Kingdom and Mineral Kingdom, A guide book to…
"Healing Yourself Holistically"!

As you have learned, it truly has made a difference in mine and my families life!

Empowering you with knowledge is the key to help you realize… that you have more power than you think !!
That Herbs and Crystals are our allies, and want to help us!

It's my passion to assist you… Heal Yourself Holistically!!

Enjoy!

DISCLAIMER

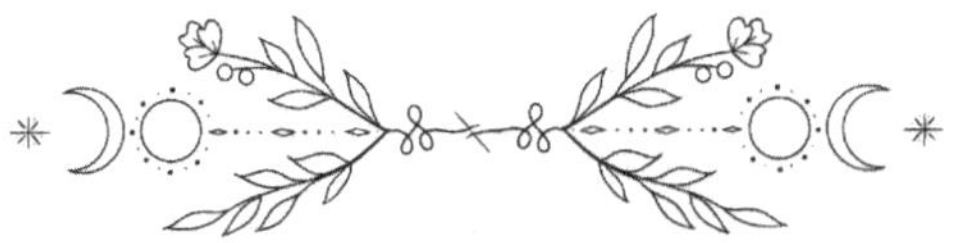

Before we dive deep into the amazing healing powers of the Plant Kingdom & Mineral Kingdom, it's important that I share with you my disclaimer!

Please use Herbs with Caution!

Some Herbs can interact with medications you are currently taking! Therefore, it's important to do your homework and make sure that before you start taking any of the Herbs listed in this book, that you double check to insure the safety for your current situation.

Feel free to consult with your Doctor before starting any of these Herbs if you have concerns. Ask your Doctor questions, and do your own research deeper into the Herb(s) of your interest.

In this book I listed as many side effects and words of caution in my "Herbal list" as I could, but still make sure you double check before taking!

For the most part, people won't experience many side effects from Herbs… but again every body is different.

Crystals are also an amazing tool for healing!
Please keep in mind, that Crystal Healing and other types of energy work are not to be considered as a substitute for conventional medicine.

If you have a serious health issue, you should consult your Doctor and make energy healing part of a compete health care program.

And as always, if you have questions….please feel free to reach out to me and I will always do my best to assist you.

~ "Heal Yourself Holistically" ~ Bridget M. Shoup ~

PREDISPOSITION

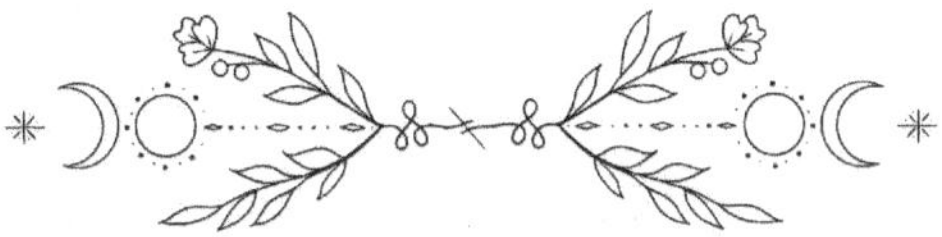

I felt it was important to cover this topic before we move on into healing yourself! The topic of Predisposition!

Question:
What is a Genetic Predisposition??

Answer:
How genetically you are susceptible to developing a particular disease.

Here is something to consider. Even though you might be genetically predisposed to a certain disease doesn't mean you will indeed get that disease!

Did you know, **only 5%** of any disease you might experience is due to a genetic predisposition!

It's true!!

That leaves 95% up to YOU!!

That is a huge deal!! It's very empowering to know!
For example, just because someone in your family might have dementia, doesn't mean YOU will!

A lot of the time YOU create your situation or disease!   You can create the type of life you live!! The Universe will expand upon whatever it is you focus your attention on. Be it good, or bad, the Universe doesn't decide…. that part is all UP TO YOU!!

How do you want your story to play out? One full of disease, sadness and pain? Or one abundant in health, wellness, happiness and joy?

Now yes, not a whole 95% is up to you, as some diseases are environmental I'll give you that.

We have all heard and seen Geoengineering, you know the lines that happen in our skies (aka chemtrails)…. it does truly affect our well-being!

Another thing we have going against that number is vaccines! Vaccine ingredients are not held to a high standard these days!

The additives are most certainly not healthy for us, including things such as aluminum, human & animal cells, mercury, latex rubber, and so so much more!

It's been known that vaccines have caused a huge spike in autism, asthma, auto immune diseases, learning disabilities, and childhood diabetes just to name a few. Not only is the issue the additives in the vaccines, but the amount these young children are receiving.

Back in 1995 a child would get 13 total vaccine doses by the age of 18 months old.

In 2016 a child would get 26 total vaccine doses by the age of 18 months old.

As you see that is a huge jump up in the total vaccines our children are "required" to be given! It's no big surprise that so much illness is haunting them at such a young age!

The sad thing is the number of recommend vaccines continues to rise each year! A child born in 2020 will receive 45 total vaccines by time they are 18 months old! Yikes!

It's important to be mindful of these things, as they also go against that 95% !

Please educate yourself on vaccines for you and your children.
I'm a pro-choice type of person and I want to educate people so they can make an informed decision!   Just know that it's your body and your choice!
Always ask questions and do your own research!

Another reason for disease in our bodies is how we are treating them!!

Imagine This…

Let's imagine for a moment that…you are a car!
In order to run for a long life and smoothly, you need to take care of yourself!

There are a few things you need to do to keep running at an optimal performance!!

One of course is the fuel!
What type of fuel are you feeding yourself (your body) ?

Are you fueling up with items that are high in fats, meats and dairy?
Or are you fueling up with veggies & fruits, and occasion meat & dairy items?

Next, is the maintenance!
Are you allowing oil changes (self love) ?
Are you rebooting with efficient sleep ?

Then we have movement!
If a car sits in a driveway for years and never moves… it won't work right anymore! Things start to seize up.

Just like your body!!
Are you moving it in ways to keep it flexible and running at it's best (exercise) ?

Moving our bodies with exercise is highly important to allow our Soul the ability to continue to play in our bodies as long as we can.

Your body is the vehicle for your Soul to drive during this life time!! Treat it right so it might continue to help you manifest your dreams and wishes.

All and all, how you decide to interact with your environment dictates your well being and health! Illness is a result of imbalances within your personal energy! Finding balance within your emotional, mental, physical & spiritual bodies is key... and will allow you to find, and continue to stay in a healthy way.

UNDERSTANDING DIS-EASE

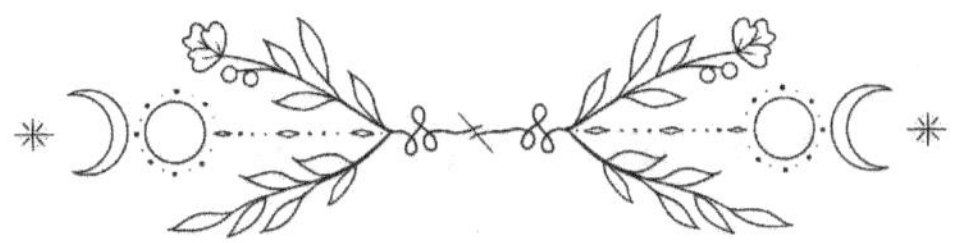

No , I didn't misspell dis-ease!
From now on in this book you will see disease referred to as dis-ease.
Let me explain why!!

Question: What is dis-ease??

Answer: Lack of ease.

Yep, it's that simple… lack of ease!

With that being said, we should be mindful to not give our power away to any aliments or dis-ease we are facing!

It's best not label it. We should recognize that what we are currently experiencing is only temporary.

As I said, when we have dis-ease, our body is not at ease.
It's not functioning properly at the moment.
The great thing is, we have the ability to flip it around.

We do this by first figuring out what has cause this dis-ease within our body in the first place.
Is it stress, anxiety, worry, or anger?
Usually those are the culprits for a lot of dis-ease.

Once we pin point what the trigger is, then we can look for the solution.

Keep in mind, we have been programmed to believe… that we need to "fix" an aliment or dis-ease with pharmaceutical drugs or vaccines.

This is NOT always the answer!

Usually that is a "band-aid" fix approach to an underlying challenge. Figure out your triggers, and then continue to find the solution that works best for you.

The best solution in my opinion of course are Herbs & Crystals! They have been on our planet for millions of years and are willing and ready to assist us!

Even better, the side effects are so minimal with Herbs & Crystals, you'll be amazed! You have the power to make any dis-ease within your body become at ease yet again!

We all want health and happiness in our life!
To have a Healthy Self, we need to first understand it starts within!
We can break it down like this…

Healthy self
HEAL THY SELF

You have the power to Heal Thy Self!!
Stay positive and keep a good outlook, realizing that as you believe in yourself and your own healing process… then you will start to see results!

It's time to take your power back, and with the support of Herbs and Crystals… you too can Heal Thy Self!!

ALTERNATIVE HEALING

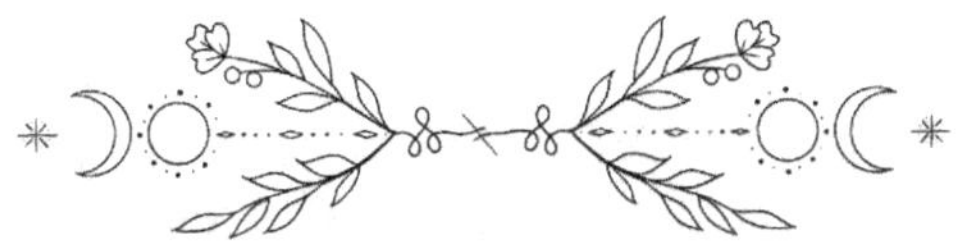

I wanted to take a moment and recognize a few other alternative healing modalities. We are so blessed with so many options!

I really do feel that some of these things have been long forgotten, but are making there reemergence !!

In addition to Herbs and Crystals as healing modalities, there are many other forms of healing that are alternative as well!

I want to cover some of them here so you know you have additional options.

Continue in the pages ahead to learn more!

Sound Healing

What is Sound Healing?
Sound healing is best way to raise your vibration!!

A Sound Healer will use things such as Bells, Crystal Singing Bowls, Tibetan Singing Bowls, Chimes, Tingshas, or even Binaural Beats (Hz frequency music) like Hemi Sync to heal the Mind, Body and Spirit.

Usually done in a group setting.
I offer Crystal Sound Healing Sessions (as I like to call them).
This is where I either go to a client's home, or I do group events where we gather.

I help get the individuals relaxed 1st with a Guided Meditation.
Following that, I will play my Crystal Singing Bowls.

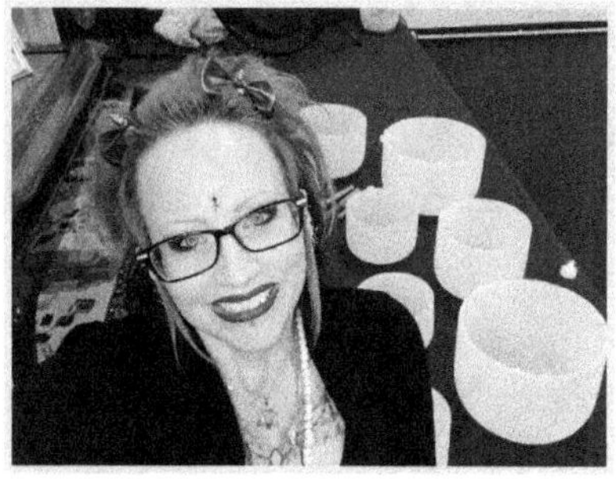

Each one of my Singing Bowls (I have 7) have a different hertz frequency that corresponds with one of the 7 Chakra's within the energetic body system.

What happens is our body is able to relax and sync up with that frequency. Which in turn allows our body to be able to heal it's self!

Leaving you feeling completely relaxed, refreshed and rejuvenated. Being in a more positive attitude as you move forward along your path.

Meditation

The reason why I picked Meditation as an alternative healing modality is because when we Meditate, we calm our mind.

Our minds are a very powerful thing!   Your mind dictates your situation. When we have a clear, calm mind, we are not only able to heal ourselves, but can see and choose a better path for ourselves

Usually we are over thinking things, and most of the time… we get carried away. Sometimes it's in a negative way too.

By practicing Meditation, you will start to notice that you can turn things around! Calming the mind is a great way to reboot your current situation. Allowing you to think before you react. As how we react to things is where our true power lies.

When we train our minds to be more quiet and calm, we are more connected to our inner-self!! By tapping into our inner-self, we will be able to pick up messages and realize why we are experiencing a dis-ease or disruption in our body.

Some benefits of Meditation are:
- Stress Reduction
- Improves Health
- Improves Sleep
- Slows Aging
- Emotional Stability
- Allows Positive Thinking
- Abundance of Happiness

It doesn't have to take long, you could honestly meditate for 5 minutes a day and still reap the benefits!

The goal is to be present in the moment, and release thought. As you notice thoughts pop into your head, see them like clouds in the sky. Allow them to blow right on by! Return your focus to your breath.
The more you practice meditation, the easier it will get to clear your mind.
Feel free to fly over to my site (www.BMoonStruck.com) to try some of my free guided meditations I offer! Click in the drop down menu "Meditation".

Visualization

Visualization is another incredible tool to have in your tool belt!

This is an excellent way to heal your Mind, Body & Spirit!
Visualization is when you actively go into a Meditative state, and you visualize in your mind's eye a positive outcome to a situation.

As we know, cancer has affected so many we love… here is an example on how to visualize the cancer away!!

For example…
Cancer is the current challenge.
Let's get more specific and say it's breast cancer.

What you would do during visualization is you would quiet your mind, go into a meditative state.

Then you would picture the tissue of your breast where the cancer is. See it, notice how it has an unhealthy look. You might see it as a color (say black). See it, what does that cancer cell look like to you? How does it feel?

Next, you would picture a white light of pure positive energy entering in through your Crown Chakra (at the top of your head) and going down and entering into your breast tissue where the cancer is.

See that white light dissolving that nasty cancer cell you saw earlier.
Watch as that black color disappears under the bright healing light.
Feel the relief and release as the cancer once and for all exits your body!
See it leave you… without a trace!

Now, see yourself completely healthy!
Enjoying life, feeling happier than before, being completely healthy.

Feel this new healthy body you get to inhabit!
Notice the happy emotion and exuberance as you carry on with your daily life, living cancer free!

Another way to do this, is to picture a pac-man like friend… entering into you body system, and eating up all the nasty cancer cells. Watch as the pac-man finds all the cancer and takes it away from you. See him exit your body and again, feel the feelings and emotions of being completely cancer free!

Do this as many times as you feel necessary (preferably daily).

<u>Affirmations</u>

Another way to set yourself up for healing success is Affirmations!
Visualization is similar to affirmations.

However, in my experience visualization is a more powerful way to manifest things for yourself.

With that being said, I still personally do affirmations each day.
(I call them spells).
Another thing you might hear affirmations being called is mantras or prayers.

An affirmation is when you make a positive statement, in order to redirect your thought process to a more successful outcome.

For example…

"I am Strong and Positive."

"I give Myself Permission to Heal."

"I am Willing to Forgive Myself."

"I Let Go of the Need to Be Right."

"I Let Go of My Perceived Pain."

"I Trust That Everything In My Life is Unfolding Perfectly."

"Everything I am Going Through is Making Me Stronger & Wiser."

The best way to do affirmations is 1st thing in the morning, or even right before bed. But you can honestly do them anytime you feel like you need a pick-me-up!

By doing affirmations these words get infused into your DNA, and as you are faced with challenges…. you will subconsciously remember that you are indeed "Strong & Positive" and it allows you a reboot before you head down a negative path.

Crystal Reiki Healing

This holistic healing modality has been around for years!!
Let's break this down.

Crystal Healing= "Laying On Of Stones".
When a Crystal Healing practitioner lays stones on a client's body in order to achieve healing and balance for the client.

Reiki= "Laying On Of Hands."
This is when a Reiki practitioner will place their hands on different parts of the client's body, channeling Life Force Energy and sharing that with the client in order to achieve healing and balance for the client.

When we combine the two
Crystal Reiki Healing= When a Crystal Reiki Master employs the use of Crystals (stones) and channels Life Force Energy in an effort to heal their client of pain or discomfort within their body, mind, spirit.

Crystal healing has been around for 6,000 years. Dating all the way back to the ancient Sumerians of Mesopotamia. Our ancient ancestors worked with Crystals in a way to achieve healing that dates all the way back to 4th millennium BC. The ancient Egyptians were also big on working with Crystals as well, and it continues in popularity today!

Reiki was developed in 1922 by a Japanese Buddhist named Mikao Usui. This method of holistic healing has been taught and passed down from Reiki Master to Reiki Master for centuries.

I personally do Crystal Reiki Healing Sessions for my Clients!
Being that I'm "The Crystal Healing Gypsy" I travel to my Client's homes and offices to offer this amazing healing service.

If you'd like an in person session, and live near me....you can always get in touch! I also offer Distant Crystal Reiki Healing Sessions!

The awesome thing is that energy healing has the ability to go beyond physical proximity! Allowing you to receive relief and detoxification within your physical, emotional, mental and spiritual bodies.

Chapter 1

WELCOME TO THE

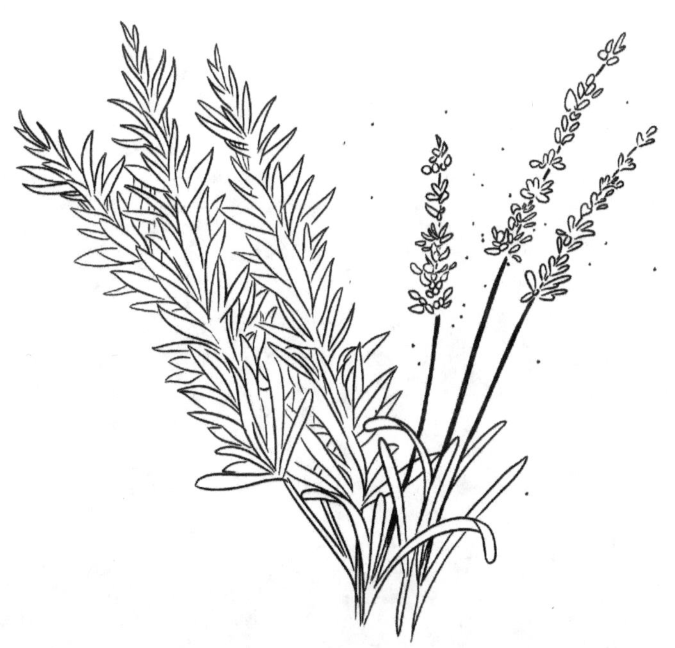

Plant Kingdom

SECTION 1
HERBAL HISTORY

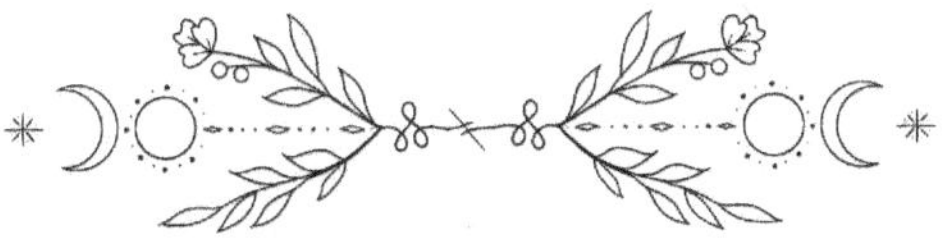

Herbalism has been around way longer than pharmaceutical drugs! In fact, a lot of the pharmaceutical drugs we have on the market today are thanks to the plants and herbs on our Earth!

For example, did you know poppies and kratom both exhibit an opioidal   type effect on the body ?   Very similar to the common drugs we have on the markets today, like Hydrocodone or Norcos.

Before the creation of pills in a lab, people would pay a visit to their local medicine man or woman.
The Witch Doctors of the time, to get the herbs to help them ease their dis-ease.

What I feel has happened is that all the old century ways of dealing with our health (the use of Herbs & Crystals) got pushed to the back of the cupboard, so to speak.

What used to be known and passed down for generations, soon was replaced by the invention of the TV, a nice little distraction.
This is where the masses got manipulated to believe what was being broadcasted…. and well, it's still going on today!

With TV ads suggesting to go to your Doctor to get a prescription for an aliment, rather than working with the lovely plant & mineral medicines we have available to us like we did in times of old.

Everyone looking for the "quick fix" instead of diving deeper into their Soul to find the real issues for their dis-ease.

It doesn't take long before it becomes the new norm, and people

started to rush out to get on the latest drugs to either help them lose weight or stop that headache.

Again, adjusting to what you're being taught… we all followed along and became almost like zombies without thinking and just ran to the Doctor for that "quick pill fix."   Thus becoming the new "norm"!

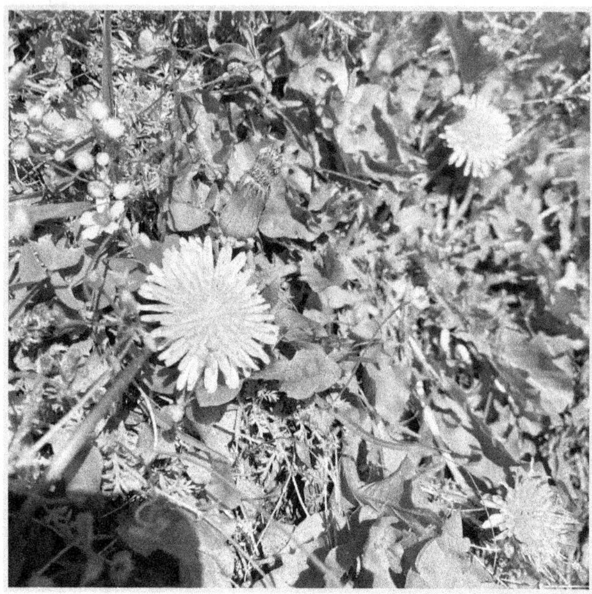

The exciting thing is.. Now people are starting to wake up and realize that they have more options than they were lead to believe.

That you need to be your own advocate and be self-reliant!
This book will hopefully help you in these ways!

So that we can appreciate the use of plants medicinally, let's explore a bit deeper into the history of herbalism!!

The use of plants as medicine actually predates humans!! Amazing right!? Evidence has been found that plant medicine was used during the Paleolithic time approximately 60,000 years ago.
Remnants of particular plant species were found in burial sites from all the way back then!

Fast forwarding… not too long ago (September 1991) the discovery of Otzi the Iceman. His body was frozen and found in the Otztal Alps after 5,000 years!! He had evidence on him of medicinal herbs. The herbs they had found on him where herbs to treat intestinal parasites.

Ancient Egypt where also really big into plant medicine. They have documentation in the "Papyrus Ebers."
The "Papyrus Ebers" lists different aliments and their treatments!

"Papyrus Ebers" dates back to 1500 BCE, they took the time to list 850 different plant medicines and their treatments.
Some of the herbs listed are Garlic, Juniper, Cannabis, Castor Bean, Aloe, and Mandrake.

Then we have ancient India where Ayurvedic medicine was born!
(Ayurveda translation: The science of life)

They are known to employ the herb Turmeric for healing, as early as 4,000 BC. Turmeric is widely used as an anti-inflammatory herb today!

China also has records dating back to the Bronze age. They have records from their emperor Shennong, where the first writings of the Chinese pharmacopoeia called "Shennong Ben Cao Jing" listed 365 medicinal plants and their uses.

In the book there are references to Ephedra, an herb that introduced Ephedrine to modern medicine. Additional mentions of herbs were Hemp and Chaulmoogra, which together where their way to curing leprosy.

Then of course I will close this section in herbal history with a mention to "The Father of Western Medicine" Hippocrates. He was a Greek physician who's collection of texts called "The Hippocratic Corpus" included recipes and remedies to heal, dating all the way back to the 5th century BC.

Hippocrates went on and shared his knowledge with others in his school "Hippocratic School of Medicine".

Some of his most famous quotes are:

"It is more important to know what sort of person has a disease than to know what sort of disease a person has." ~Hippocrates

"If we could give every individual the right amount of nourishment and exercise, not too little and not too much, we would have found the safest way to health." ~Hippocrates

"The natural healing force within each of us is the greatest force in getting well." ~Hippocrates

I absolutely love that Hippocrates understood that we can heal ourselves. Of course with the use of Herbs and Minerals, we most certainly can help our bodies along the way.

As you read this book, keep in mind that your body can truly heal its self!
It's a matter of mind set, and what you are fueling your body with… and what type of activity you decide to spend your time on makes a difference.

Once you understand these things, you will start to recognize life altering transformations happen for you.

Everything is good with balance. Working with Herbs as a way to heal yourself naturally… is one of the best things you can do, to give yourself that extra assistance in healing.

~ "Heal Yourself Holistically" ~ Bridget M. Shoup ~

SECTION 2
EXPIRATION DATES & STORAGE

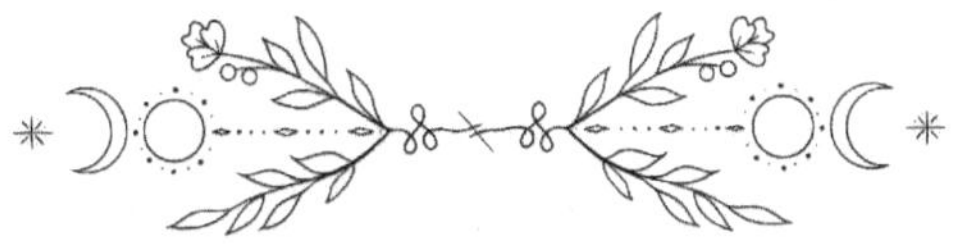

Have you ever wondered about the expiration dates on your herbal supplements or vitamins?

Have you gotten prescriptions and noticed an expiration on them?

Are they still good?
Can I still take them??
Will they be as effective???

Well, this chapter is going to cover all these questions and so much more!!

As it turns out, the "expiration dates" on bottles aren't what you think!   In 1979 drug manufactures were required to place an expiration date on their products.   They had to spend money and time to test their products to come to that date on the bottle.

BUT,
That date is not an expiration date, it's a guarantee of the products full potency.

There has been documentation of the FDA (Food & Drug Administration) conducting a test, as per request from the US military on their stock pile of drugs.

The test conduced that 90% of more than 100 drugs tested (prescription & over the counter drugs) were perfectly good to use.
Even after their expiration dates… which was of that 15 years pass the stamped date, when the test was concluded !

This just goes to show that the expiration date doesn't really indicate a point in which the medication or supplements is   no longer effective or has become unsafe for use.

Of course 10% of the drugs they tested where NOT ok to take after their expiration date. Some of the drugs that are not recommend to take past the expiration date are drugs like nitroglycerine, insulin, and liquid antibiotics.

So there you have it, most drugs and supplements are safe to take after the stamped expiration date!!

Nice thing is it will probably help save you some money if you have these herbs in the back of your cupboard and its's been a while!

When you look at your herb cabinet, you might be wondering now… well how long will my herbs last, if there is no expiration date listed?

As a rule of thumb, most herbs will last about 3 years.
If you have a spice or herb that is whole, about 4 years.
Ground herbs and spices, 2-3 years.
Dried herbs, about 1-3 years.

Storage is everything!!
How you store your herbs matter!
It will play a big part into how long they will last!

Some tips:

- Store in a cool dark cupboard
- Store AWAY from direct heat or sunlight
- Keep in a tightly closed bottle
- Visual test (if it looks bad, toss it)
- Smell test (if it smells bad, toss it)

If you're like me, you like to grow your own herbs!
I have an abundance of my all time favorite, Rosemary!

What I do is a few times a year, I will harvest my Rosemary.
Wash it, hang it up to dry (depending on the temp usually takes about 3-4 weeks)…. and then I use my mortar and pestle to grind up the herbs.

Next I place them in a glass container with a screw on lid, making it easy and accessible when I'm baking or cooking to grab a pinch here and there to liven up my meals! This is another great way to work with the healing energies of Herbs!

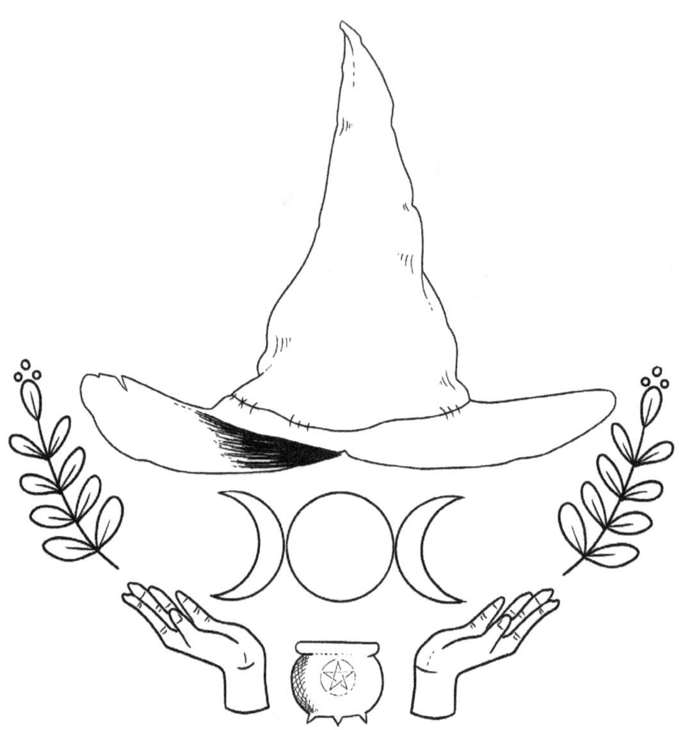

SECTION 3
MAGICKAL HERBS
(FOR *WITCHES*)

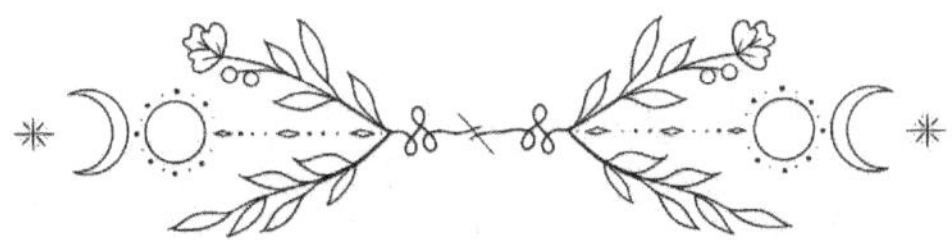

I decided to include this portion in my book, some magickal knowledge if your into witchcraft like me!

I wanted this herbal book to have the best of both worlds!! So if you are not into this type of thing, it's ok.
I do feel that if you go into this subject with an open mind, you just might learn something interesting and new in this section.

I felt having a book on herbs needed to include the magickal working with them, as I personal work with herbs for both medicinal and magickal purposes! An easy and convenient way to have all the info. in one place!

Let's take a moment to define Magick !

Magick: *The practice of causing change through the use of powers as yet not defined or accepted by science.*
The "k" in Magick is an indication that you are working with the powers within you to make this said change.
Usually with the assistance of Plants, Crystals, Candles, Elements and so forth.

When we do spell work, it's usually to obtain a different outlook to a situation. Some reasons for magickal workings would be protection, love, positivity, calmness, healing, etc.

One thing to keep in mind is when we do our Magick, we do the spells and then let them go! You don't need to think about it, allow the magick to bake within the belly of the Universe. It's the Universe's job to expand upon our magickal askings. All we have to do is stay in a high vibration, one of positive emotions.

If you think about it, it's just like baking a cake. When we put the cake into the oven, you don't open the door several times to check on it to make sure it's doing it's job? No! You simply trust and know that you put the work in and a positive outcome will follow.

Consider this when doing your Magickal Spell work. Do your spells and then let them go, trusting in the Universal energies to follow up with the positive outcome!

Before we begin, let me say… I identify as a Solitary Eclectic Witch.
I don't associate with any one religion.
I practice different types of witchcraft, and have come up with a combination that feels right to me!
That's the best part of being a Witch, you get to pick and choose your own personalized path!

I believe in Divine energy and that everything on this planet has a spirit!
Yes, I'm that lady who will find a spider, bee, or cricket in the house… pick it up and release it in my backyard! And Yes, it totally freaks out my Daughter!

Plants are the same!! They have their own special spirit! When we do harvest live herbs, it's important to thank them for their assistance and sacrifice . I always make sure to do this verbally and place my hands on them and ask if it's ok that I partake. I feel that is very important to share!

As with Herbs being different, each Witch practices differently as well. These of course are my ideas in this section. I will list different herbs I enjoy working with in my practice and their best applications. If you work with these Herbs differently in your practice, that's great!! It's always good to experiment and figure out what works best for you! Another perk to being a Witch, there are no concrete rules!

I can say for certain, there is one thing I know that most all Witches who practice follow in common …
that is the rule of "Harm None"!

In addition to that rule, I personally follow "The Rule of 3" which is… anything you do comes back to you three fold. Therefore, I only do spells and magickal working that reflect positivity in mine and other's life's.

Side note: It's always best to check with someone before doing a spell on their behalf.

Other Magickal Rules:
- Harm none.. not even yourself!
- Magick can be used as a defense, but never for attacks.
- Magick is love, all Magick should be done with love.
- Magick required effort… you get what you put in.
- Magick is natural.

I will be covering the use of Herbs for magickal purposes here. Some of the most popular ones and how to work with herbs to amp up your spell work!

So… with a wave of my wand, off we go!

As we have learned earlier in this book, there is a long history in Herbs for medicinal reasons.

But, what you might not be aware of is that herbs also have a long history in a witchy ritual sense as well!

In Greek mythology, we know that Hecate (the patroness of Witches) taught her daughters the herbal arts! Just like the times of old, things were passed down from Witch to Witch… generation to generation.

In the 1400's there was an Italian Witch named Matteuccia Francisco. She perfected the craft of working with Herbs for magical workings and was found mixing over 30 plant parts into wine for love, fertility or other type things.

Matteuccia was so well versed in plant lore, and adeptness with the magickal arts that she even had clients that would travel from hundreds of miles to work with her.

Each Herb carries it's own special characteristics and magickal properties.
We are so blessed to have the ability to not only heal with these magnificent Herbs, but to also make magick happen for ourselves with them!

Many Witches, whether be it Pagan, Wiccan, or no religious association… have worked with herbs as part of their regular magickal ritual practice.

Herbs for magickal uses are quite vast!
Protection, Purification, Healing, Strength, Health, Money, Success or for Beauty…yep, there's an herb for that!

So let's dive into some of my favorite herbs that I work with for Magickal purposes and how you can work with them to!

<u>Sage</u>

Most people, especially Witches love Sage!!
Sage is known to have the ability to disinfect, protect and remove negative energy! Visit any Witches house and you will see & smell billowing clouds of Sage smoke, as a Witch's top priority is to maintain a cleansed space!

◆ *Stats:*
Gender: Masculine
Element: Air
Planet: Jupiter

◆ *Magickal Use:*
Carry a leaf of Sage in your wallet to attract money & wealth.

◆ *Witchy Properties:*
Cleansing, Protection, Purification, Wisdom, Health, Exorcism, Wish Magick, Emotional Strength, Healing Grief, Banish Nightmares.

◆ *Medicinal Properties:*
Increases Memory, Eases Digestion, Calms Anxiety, Increases Mental Performance, Reduces High Cholesterol, Treats Cold Sores, Reduces Menopausal Symptoms.

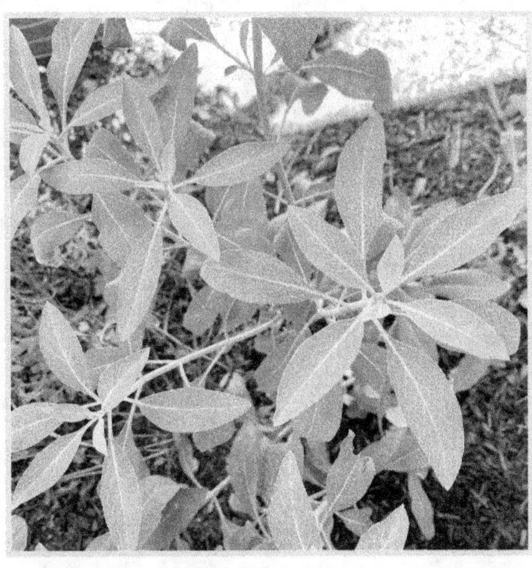

Lavender

Another popular herb, this lovely little purple flower with it's soothing smell has been captivating people for centuries! This is one of my favorites in my witch herb cabinet. I love also working with Lavender in my Crystal Grid workings!

◆ *Stats:*
Gender: Masculine
Element: Air
Planet: Mercury

◆ *Magickal Use:*
Place some dried Lavender buds in a sachet bag and place in your pillow for sweet dreams.

◆ *Witchy Properties:*
Attraction & Beauty Spells, Cleansing Spells, Healing & Longevity, Love Spells, Increasing Intelligence, Sleep, Removal of Harmful Energies, Communication with Spirits, Promotes Clarity of Thought & Generates Visions.

◆ *Medicinal Properties:*
Relieves Stress, Accelerates the Healing Process, Great for Burns and Bug Bites, Treats Anxiety, Depression, Insomnia, Relaxes Stomachache and Nausea, Prevents Hair loss, Relieves Pain from Sprains and Muscle Soreness.

Rosemary

Something that I personally grow in my backyard is Rosemary!   I absolutely love it's smell, it's so revitalizing!!   I enjoy adding some of my dried Rosemary to dress my candles, when I do candle magick! Another great way I incorporate this lovely herb is by placing pinches of it in my cooking (yep, I'm a bit of a kitchen Witch too).

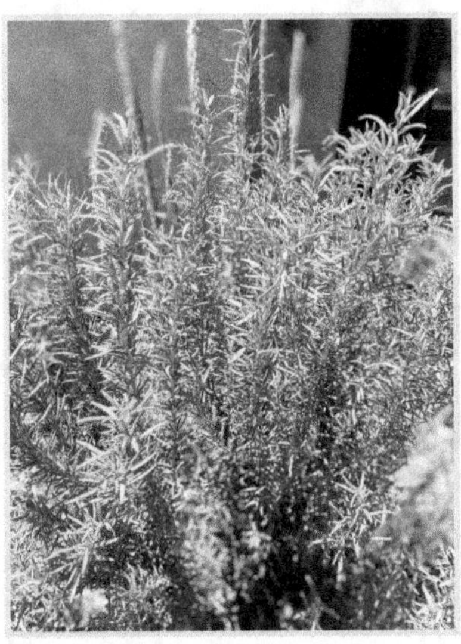

◆*Stats:*
Gender: Masculine
Element: Fire
Planet: Sun

◆*Magickal Use:*
Pick your favorite essential oil and rub on a candle of your choice. Apply the Rosemary by rolling the candle in the herb. This will be a dressing to your candle adding the witchy properties to your spell! Super when doing candle magick! Great for any type of Witch Craft.

◆ *Witchy Properties:*
Love, Romance, Healing & Purification, Protection, Consecrating, Blessing, Vitality, Wisdom, Mental Powers, Youth.

◆ *Medicinal Properties:*
Boosts Immune System, Relieves Sore Throats, Great for Promoting Hair Growth, Clears Up your Complexion, Soothes Eczema, Boosts Memory.

Star Anise

Also known as Anise Estrella, these cute little star like herbs are a Witches favorite for sure! Not only for it's benefits, but for it's yummy smell! Throwing a few into your fire place is a great way to add a little magick into your hearth.

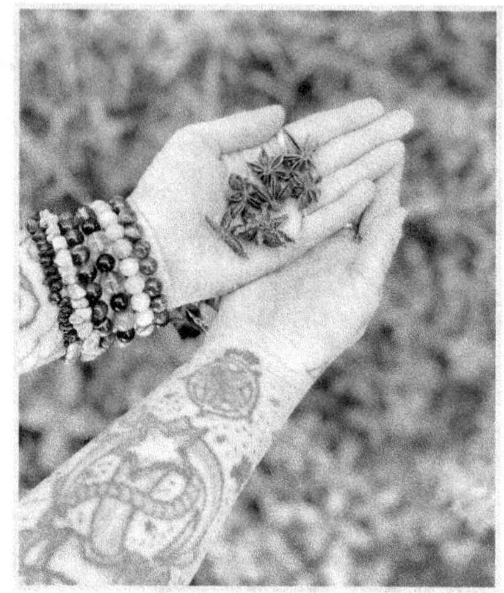

◆ *Stats:*
Gender: Masculine
Element: Air
Planet: Jupiter

✦ *Magickal Use:*
During your New Moon Ritual, burn this lovely herb as you are connecting with your Spirit Guides, or doing any type of divination work.

✦ *Witchy Properties:*
Increases Psychic Awareness, Protection from Evil Eye, Good Luck, Induces Calm, Enhances Clairvoyance, Great for Protection During Travel.

✦ *Medicinal Properties:*
Great as a Digestive Aid, Gas Relief, Natural Flu Fighter, Kills Bacteria, Boosts Appetite, Lowers the Risk of Cancer.

Mugwort

This herb is one of the most popular among the Witches! Amazing for helping enhance clairvoyance, this herb was used back in the day to keep beer fresh (before they discovered hops).

◆ *Stats:*
Gender: Feminine
Element: Earth
Planet: Venus

◆ *Magickal Use:*
Prepare Mugwort as a tea to aid during divination and scrying. Highly connected to the Lunar Cycle and the Crone. Great to incorporate during New/Full Moon Ritual workings.

◆ *Witchy Properties:*
Beneficial in Scrying work, Divination, Helps with Lucid Dreaming, Increases Psychic Ability, Strength, Astral Projection, Great to work with Lunar Magick, Protection.

◆ *Medicinal Properties:*
Disinfectant type properties, Anxiety, Depression & Stress relief, Insect Repellant, Treats Gas, Diarrhea and Constipation, Headaches, Fever, Nerve Issues, Insomnia.

Basil

Most people have heard of this herb! Basil is used in lots of Italian type recipes. Not only is it a yummy ingredient in your food, but it's also equally as tasty in your spell workings!

◆ *Stats:*
Gender: Masculine
Element: Fire
Planet: Mars

◆ *Magickal Use:*
Write on your basil leaf what you wish to release from your life! Light a candle, take hold of the stem of the Basil, and precede to light the leaf with the flame of the fire. As you release say aloud:
"I now remove these things from my life now… for my highest good & for the highest good of all concerned."

◆ *Witchy Properties:*
Protection Spells, Blessings, Love, Abundance, Exorcism, Money and Happiness.

◆ *Medicinal Properties:*
Helps Digestion, Depression, Diabetes Management, Anti-Inflammatory, Treats IBD/IBS, Arthritis, Fever, Headaches, Sore Throat, Cough, Cold, Flu.

~ "Heal Yourself Holistically" ~ Bridget M. Shoup ~

SECTION 4
HEALING WITH HERBS

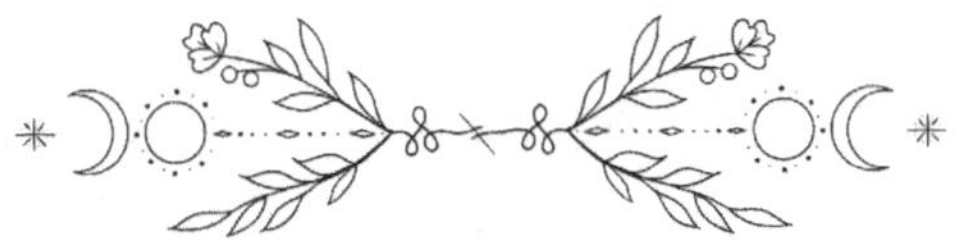

This chapter you will discover all the amazing Herbs that you can work with to assist you in the healing process!

This list is of course, not a full list with every ailment or every herb you could encounter. I wanted to cover the top ailments that most people I know are dealing with… or ones that my family and I have worked with!

As a general rule of thumb, if you are pregnant or nursing… please do you research to make sure these herbs are safe for you. Ask you Doctor! It's best to be on the side of caution when pregnancy is involved!

Remember that every body is different, it's best to start slow & when giving these herbs a try. Usually there are multiple herbs for the same ailment. This is super beneficial, for as if you find one not working as you hoped…. you can try alternative ones until you find your right fit!

You should be able to find these Herbs at your local health food stores. I like to get mine from "Sprouts", as I know they are a trusted source… plus the people who work in the vitamin department are quite knowledgeable if you have additional questions about the herb.

Another place to pick up Herbs are online!
A few of my favorites are "Mountain Rose Herbs" and "Swanson".

"Mountain Rose Herbs" (www.mountinroseherbs.com) is great for when your looking for loose herbs. Perfect for making your own teas or for spell workings.

"Swanson" (www.swansonvitamins.com) also has high quality herbs, ready for your consumption in capsules or tincture form.

I should note…. I'm <u>not</u> affiliated with "Mountain Rose Herbs", "Swanson", or "Sprouts"… it's just my recommendation.

As always, use your best judgment when purchasing your Herbs… you always want the highest of quality!

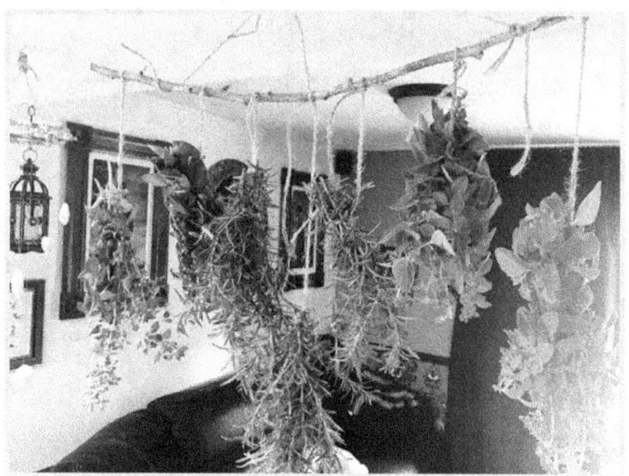

An alternative way of working with Herbs are to of course, grow your own!

One of the easiest Herbs I have found that grows really well is Rosemary & Aloe Vera! There are so many others too!! I have also had success in growing Lemon Balm (which is great if you suffer from insomnia).

➥Different Form Of Herbs:
Tablets, Capsules, Tinctures, Teas, Powders

Tablets & Capsules
These two are pretty much the same, usually the herbal supplement company will have the Herbs pressed in a tablet form.
The most common is the capsule, which is usually made of a gel that will dissolve in your stomach.   This capsule has the herbs inside them.

Tinctures
This is the liquid form of taking a Herbal supplement. This is the concentrated version of the Herb where they extract it's Herbal content by soaking the bark, berries, leaves or roots. Then is added to an alcohol or vinegar to help pull out the active ingredients and help it from spoiling.

Teas
Most people are familiar with tea! Quite common in the UK, tea drinking is quite beneficial! You can add your favorite loose Herbs in a tea ball or bag and allow their amazing healing energy to come through. Adding them to a warm cup of water and steeping for at least 10 minutes. Then enjoy! Of course, the longer your steep, the stronger the tea will be!

Powders
Sometimes you will find the Herbs in a powder form. It's best to use these by mixing them into food or drink. Another thing you could do is purchase capsules and fill them yourself!

Which ever is your method of taking Herbs, it's all good! As always, It's best to find what works for you.

A Word of Caution:

If you are already taking prescription drugs, it's best to check with your Doctor/Pharmacist before starting Herbal supplements.

Certain Herbs may interfere with the strength of your current prescription drugs.

You could also have an adverse effect when taking certain prescriptions together with Herbs.

Always do your homework to make sure it's safe for you and your current situation.

I have done my best to list some possible side effects and or interactions… but again, double check before starting!

Also, you will notice I list numerous Herbs per ailment. You do not need to take all the Herbs listed, just pick one you'd like to try and see how it works for you.

Every body is different and therefore, different Herbs might work better for your bodily chemical makeup than others.
So, try one of the Herbs listed and if it isn't achieving the affects you where hoping for… then move on and try one of the other Herbal options listed.

My Herbal List is in alphabetical order based on the ailment.
You might notice a lot of the same Herbs are used for many ailments!

At the back of the book in the index, I will list the Herbs by name and it's page number so you can reference all the ailments that particular Herb will assist with.

Enjoy exploring the Herbal Kingdom!!
So… let's get onward with the list!!

Herbal List

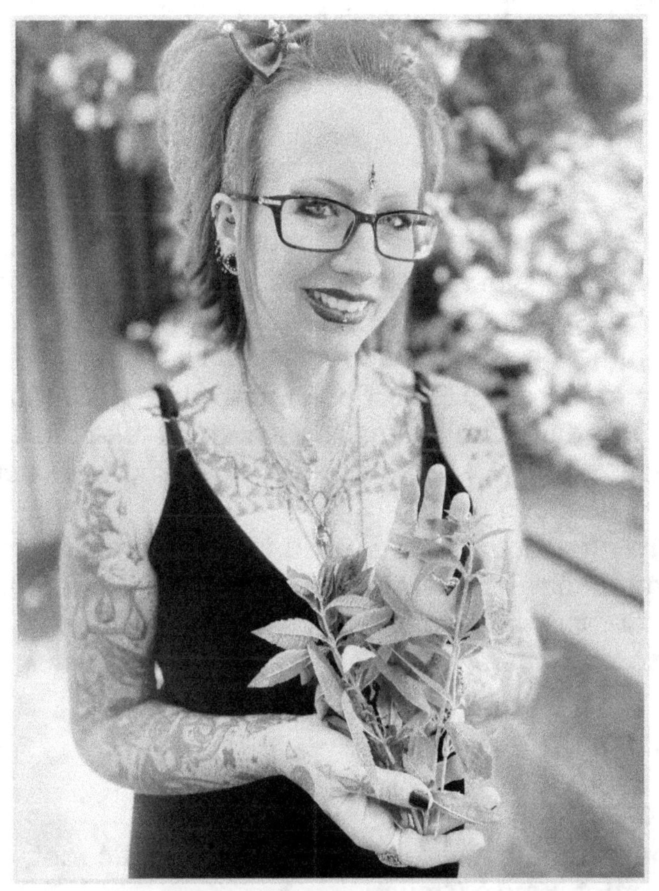

To Assist You In The Healing Process!

-A-

<u>ADHD</u>
Other Herbs To Try: Gaba, Rhodiola rosea, Fish Oil, Vitamin B-Complex (B6 Vitamins)

Gaba
- ✦ **Other Names:** Gamma-aminbutyric acid
- ✦ **Use:** Depression, Stress, Anxiety, Has a calming effect, Improves sleep, relieves symptoms of PMS, Decreases inflammation, improves focus in ADHD.
- ✦ **How to Take:** Capsule, Tablet, Lozenges 250-400 mg. 3x's per day. Take in small doses, don't take too often only as needed, start with lower dose and work your way up as needed.
- ✦ **Warnings:** Not recommended for pregnant or nursing women, may interact with meds for anxiety, depression or insomnia, if you have skin tinging or flushing... discontinue use.

Rhodiola rosea
- ✦ **Other Names:** r.rosea, Golden Root, Arctic root, Roseroot, King's Crown
- ✦ **Use:** Helps improve physical and mental energy, brain boosting, Reduces stress, improving stamina, fights depression, supports weight loss helps burn off belly fat.
- ✦ **How to Take:** Capsule or tablet, or tea 250-700 mg. day. Take 15 mins. before meals.
- ✦ **Warnings:** can cause temporary dizziness & dry mouth. If these persist, stop taking.

ALLERGIES

Other Herbs To Try: Stinging Nettle, Butterbur, Garlic, Rosemary, Turmeric

Stinging Nettle

- ✦ **Other Names:** Urtica dioica, Nettle Leaf, Nettle
- ✦ **Use:** Hay fever (allergic rhinitis), Urinary issues like UTI, Benign prostatic hyperplasia, joint pain, sprain & strains, insect bites.
- ✦ **How to Take:** Capsule, tea, extract, creams
- ✦ **Warnings:** Can cause stomach issues, urinary issues, sweating, diarrhea, rash, Not for use in young children, if your pregnant or nursing you should not take! May interact with blood thinners, treatments for high blood pressure, heart disease medications and diabetes medications.

Butterbur

- ✦ **Other Names:** Petasites hybridus
- ✦ **Use:** Asthma, bronchitis, excess mucus (as effective as Zyrtec), Relives migraines, Reduces asthma symptoms, promotes healthy heart, decrease inflammation
- ✦ **How to Take:** capsule, tablet, or tea. 50-75 mg. 2x's per day. Begin small & increase as needed.
- ✦ **Warnings:** Not for use in young children, if your pregnant or nursing you should not take! Avoid if you have liver issues, If you allergic to ragweed, daisies, marigolds & chrysanthemums possible allergic reactions could happen. Could cause headache, diarrhea, fatigue, belching and itchy eyes.

ALZHEIMER'S

Other Herbs To Try: Ginkgo Biloba, Butterbur, Ginseng, Berberine, CoQ10, Rosemary Essential Oil, Ashwagandha

Ginkgo Biloba

✦ **Other Names:** Ginkgo, Gingko, Maidenhair Tree
✦ **Use:** Improves brain function, Slows progression of Alzheimer's, Leg cramps, Dementia, Depression, Eczema, Memory loss, Tinnitus, Asthma, Improves Circulation
✦ **How to Take:** Capsule or Tablet. It takes about 2 weeks to see results.
✦ **Warnings:** Should not be taken by people who have bleeding disorders. Stop use if having a surgery type procedures.

Ginseng

✦ **Other Names:** Panax quinquefolius, American Ginseng, P. ginseng
✦ **Use:** Improves memory, Enhances immune function, Stimulates appetite, Bronchitis, Circulatory issues, diabetes, Lack of Energy, Stress
✦ **How to Take:** Capsule or Tablet.
✦ **Warnings:** Do not take if you have high blood pressure or are pregnant/nursing.

ANEMIA

Other Herbs To Try: Moringa, Dandelion Root

Moringa
- ✦ **Other Names:** moringa oleifera
- ✦ **Use:** Anemia, Inflammation related diseases, Cancer, Diabetes, Low energy, Arthritis, Allergies, Asthma, Stomach pains, Epilepsy, High blood pressure, Kidney Stones, Thyroid Disorder, Low sex drive, Bacterial/ Fungal, Viral/Parasitic Infections.
- ✦ **How to Take:** Capsule, Tablet or tea
- ✦ **Warnings:** Don't take if your having low blood pressure issues, will temporarily interfere with fertility.

ANXIETY

Other Herbs To Try: Ashwagandha, Bupleurum, Gaba, Kava Root, Holy Basil, Skullcap, Kratom, Chamomile, Magnesium, Vitamin B Complex

Ashwagandha

✦ **Other Names:** Withania somnifera
✦ **Use:** Prevents stress, anxiety, depression, increases physical endurance, improves sexual function, Helps stabilize mood/emotions, Anti-aging, Anti-inflammatory, Stimulates immune system, Boosts Memory.
✦ **How to Take:** Capsule, Tablet, Tincture
✦ **Warnings:** N/A

Bupleurum

✦ **Other Names:** Bupleurum chinense, Bupleurum americanum, Bupleurum falcatum, Chai hu, Thorowax root, Hare's ear root, Saiko
✦ **Use:** Treats depression, improves liver function, prevents cirrhosis & liver cancer, boosts adrenal gland funciton, fights ovarian cancer, Epilepsy, PTSD
✦ **How to Take:** Capsule, Tablet, Tea
✦ **Warnings:** Could produce increased bowl moments & gas, Avoid if pregnant/nursing, Not recommended if you have a bleeding disorder, diabetes, or autoimmune disease. Stop taking 2 weeks before any surgical procedures.

ARTHRITIS

Other Herbs To Try: Cat's Claw, Ginger, Stinging Nettle, Turmeric, Boswellia, Skullcap, Evening Primrose, Noni, Holy Basil, Borage, Bromelain, Gulcosamine, Celery Seed, MSM, Fish Oil, Vitamin B6

Cat's Claw
- ✦ **Other Names:** Uncaria tomentosa, una de gato
- ✦ **Use:** Anti-inflammatory, Manages Arthritis, Stimulates immune system, Cleansing intestinal tract, Viral infections, Helps with: Cancer, Tumors, Ulcers
- ✦ **How to Take:** Capsule, Tablet
- ✦ **Warnings:** Do not use while pregnant/nursing

Ginger
- ✦ **Other Names:** Zingiber officinale
- ✦ **Use:** Anti-Inflammatory, Reduces cramps, Arthritis, Fever, Headache, Good for IBD/IBS, Hot Flashes, Indigestion, Morning Sickness, Motion Sickness, Muscle Pain, Nausea, Vomiting
- ✦ **How to Take:** Capsule, Tablet, Tincture, Tea
- ✦ **Warnings:** If taken in large quantities can cause stomach upset. Not recommended for people who take anticoagulants or have gallstones. Not recommended for extended use during pregnancy.

ASTHMA

Other Herbs To Try: Ginseng, Astragalus, Butterbur, Echinacea, Vitamin D, Magnesium

Astragalus

- ✦ **Other Names:** Astragalus membranaceus, huang qi
- ✦ **Use:** Effective for chronic lung weakness, Helps with digestion, Increases Metabolism, Promotes Healing, Increase Stamina, Fights off colds/flus
- ✦ **How to Take:** Capsule, Tablet
- ✦ **Warnings:** Do not use if fever is present

AUSTISM

Other Herbs To Try: Poria Cocos, Panax ginseng, Acorus gramineus, Schisandra chinensis, Glycyrrhiza uralensis

Panax ginseng

- ✦ **Other Names:** P. ginseng, Asian Ginseng
- ✦ **Use:** Improves normal behavior, Improves Calmness, Enhances Memory, Reduces Ulcers, Regulates Blood Glucose Levels Relieves Stress, Mental Balance, Erectile Dysfunction
- ✦ **How to Take:** Tea, Capsule
- ✦ **Warnings:** Not Recommend while pregnant/nursing. May cause drowsiness, Long term use could cause headaches, dizziness, stomaches. May affect blood sugar levels be careful if taking diabetic meds. May interfere in blood clotting. Talk to Dr. if taking meds for antidepressant, stimulants, Morphine or Antipsychotic meds.

-B-

BACTERIAL INFECTION
Other Herbs To Try: Berberine

Berberine
- ✦ **Other Names:** berberine hydrochloride
- ✦ **Use:** Bacteria infection, Metabolic Syndrome, Diabetes, Heart disease, High cholesterol, Hypertension (High blood pressure), Joint problems, Low bone density, Weight control, Depression, Sibo, Lung Inflammation, Cancer, Alzheimer's Disease, Anti-Aging
- ✦ **How to Take:** Capsule, Tablet
- ✦ **Warnings:** If taking an antibiotic or meds to lower blood sugar talk to Dr. before taking, This will lower blood pressure beware if taking meds to lower blood pressure, Not recommenced if pregnant/nursing. Some people many have cramping, diarrhea, constipation (take smaller dosages to reduce the likelihood of this issues)

BIPOLAR DISORDER

Other Herbs To Try: St. John's Wort, Holy Basil, Ashwagandha, Ginseng, Rhodiola rosea, Fish Oil

St. John's Wort
- ✦ **Other Names:** Hypericum perforatum
- ✦ **Use:** Depression, Nerve pain, Stress, Aids in wound healing, ADHD
- ✦ **How to Take:** Capsule, Tablet
- ✦ **Warnings:** May increase sensitivity to sunlight. Some people many experience gastrointestinal issues & headaches. Not recommend If taking antidepressants, birth control pills or anticoagulants.

Holy Basil
- ✦ **Other Names:** Ocimum tenuiflorum, Ocimum sanctum
- ✦ **Use:** Balances stress hormones, Fights skin infections & Acne, Controls blood glucose, Fights Cancer, Relives Fever, Improves respiratory disorder, Relieves Headaches
- ✦ **How to Take:** Capsule, Tablet, Tea
- ✦ **Warnings:** When used for an extended amount of time could cause nausea, indigestion and changes in certain hormones. Recommend to take for about 6 weeks, then take a break. Not recommend If your taking meds for blood clots or if Pregnant/Nursing.

<u>BLOOD PRESSURE</u> (See Hypertension)

<u>BOOST MEMORY</u> (See Alzheimers)

<u>BURSITS</u>
Other Herbs To Try: Turmeric, Glucosamine, Bromelian

-C-

CANCER

Other Herbs To Try: Soursop, Galangal, Skullcap, Kava, Basil, Bay Leaf, Black Currant, Boswellia, Cardamom, Cat's Claw, Thyme, Cordycep, Turmeric, Reishi Mushrooms, Vitamin B12, Vitamin D3, Ginger

Soursop
- ✦ **Other Names:** graviola, guyabano
- ✦ **Use:** Fights Cancer, Reduces Eye Disease, Anti-Inflammatory, Kills Pancreatic Cancer Cells, Treats Infections, Herpes, Cough, Vomiting
- ✦ **How to Take:** Capsule, Tea, Fruit, Tincture,
- ✦ **Warnings:** Not recommended if Pregnant/Nursing

Galangal
- ✦ **Other Names:** Alpinia galanga, Alpinia officinarum
- ✦ **Use:** Cancer Fighting, Anti-Inflammatory, Gastric Cancer, Leukemia, Melanoma, Pancreatic Cancer, Colon Cancer, Breast Cancer, Liver Cancer, Bile Duct Cancer (cholangiocarcinoma), Improves Sperm Count, Antibacterial, AntiFungal , Supports Good Brain Health, Stomachaches, Digestive Issues
- ✦ **How to Take:** Capsule, Tincture, Tea
- ✦ **Warnings:** Not Recommended if Pregnant, Consuming high doses can cause stomach upset, diarrhea and low energy

CHOLESTEROL (HIGH)

Other Herbs To Try: Hawthorne, Berberine, Ginger Root, Milk Thistle, Turmeric, Thyme, Garlic, Fish Oil, CoQ10

Hawthorne
- ✦ **Other Names:** Crataegus laevigata
- ✦ **Use:** Lowers Blood Pressure, Lowers Cholesterol levels, Anemia, Restores Heart Muscle, Boosts Immune System.
- ✦ **How to Take:** Capsule, Tea, Tincture
- ✦ **Warnings:** Do not use if you take medication for heart disease

Milk Thistle
- ✦ **Other Names:** Silybum marianum, Mary Thistle, Wild Artichoke
- ✦ **Use:** Liver disease, Kidney, Gallbladder, Adrenal disorders, IBD/IBS, Psoriasis, Weakened Immune System, Upset Stomach, Prostate & Breast Cancer, Lowers Cholesterol
- ✦ **How to Take:** Capsule, Tablet, Tincture
- ✦ **Warnings:** N/A

CONSTIPATION

Other Herbs To Try: Slippery Elm, Psyllium Husk, Triphala, Magnesium, Flaxseed oil, Chia Seeds, Aloe Vera, Chicory Root

Slippery Elm

✦ **Other Names:** Ulmus rubra, Moose Elm, Red Elm
✦ **Use:** Soothes inflamed mucous membranes, Bowels, Stomach, Urinary Tract, Diarrhea, Ulcers, Colds, Flu, Sore Throat, Crohn's Disease, IBD/IBS, Ulcerative Colitis, Diverticulosis, Gastritis
✦ **How to Take:** Capsule, Tea
✦ **Warnings:** Take 1 hour before eating. Not recommended to take long term, as it will not allow your intestines to absorb nutrients properly. May slow the absorption of drugs, take 2 hrs. away from other medications.

Psyllium Husk

✦ **Other Names:** Plantago ovata, Ispaghula
✦ **Use:** Natural Laxative, Promotes Heart Disease, Diabetes, Cancer, Colitis, Crohn's, Constipation, Diarrhea, Diverticulosis, Hemorrhoids, Hypertension, IBS, Kidney Stones, Ulcers, PMS, Lowers Cholesterol
✦ **How to Take:** Capsule, Tablet, Tincture
✦ **Warnings:** Make sure to drink enough water when taking, Not Recommended if you have esophageal narrowing or swallowing difficulties or bowel obstructions. Do not take within 1-2 hours of other prescription medications.

COMMON COLD

Other Herbs To Try: Elderberry, Black Currant, Ginger, Garlic, Echinacea, Zinc, Oregano Oil, Vitamin D

Elderberry
✦ **Other Names:** Elder, Sambucus nigra, Black Elder, Black Elderberry, European Elder
✦ **Use:** Inflammation, Cough, Colds, Flu, Congestion, Boosts Immune System, Lowers Fever, Soothes Respiratory Tract, Stimulates circulation
✦ **How to Take:** Capsule, Tea, Tincture
✦ **Warnings:** Not Recommended if Pregnant/Nursing

Black Currant
✦ **Other Names:** Ribes nigrum
✦ **Use:** Cold Symptoms, Viruses, Bacteria, Influenza H, Pylori, Whooping Cough, Cancer prevention, Heart Health, Diabetes, Prevents Glaucoma, Boost Immune System, Herpes
✦ **How to Take:** Capsule, Tablet
✦ **Warnings:** Could cause allergic reactions if you are sensitive to salicylates, Some people may experience gas, headaches, diarrhea, Not Recommend if taking phenothiazines (anti-psychoitc meds), Talk to Dr. if taking Warfain as Black Currant will slow blood clotting

<u>COUGH</u>

Other Herbs To Try: Mullein, Marshmallow Root, Slippery Elm, Asafoetida, Elderberry, Licorice Root, Ginger Root, Honey, Vitamin C, Zinc Lozenges

Mullein
- ✦ **Other Names:** Verbascum thapsus, Mullein Leaf
- ✦ **Use:** Congestion, Asthma, Bronchtitis, Difficulties Breathing, Laxative, Pain Killer, Sleep Aid, Earache, Hay Fever, Swollen Glands, Kidney Issues, Cough, Constipation, Gout
- ✦ **How to Take:** Capsule, Tea, Powder, Tincture
- ✦ **Warnings:** N/A

Marshmallow Root
- ✦ **Other Names:** Althaea officinalis
- ✦ **Use:** Helps expel mucus & fluid, Cough, Heals skin, Bladder Infections, Digestive upset, Fluid Retention, Headache, Intestinal disorders, IBD/IBS, Crohn's, Colitis, Kidney Problems, Sinusitis, Sore Throat
- ✦ **How to Take:** Capsule, Tablet
- ✦ **Warnings:** Take for 4 weeks, then take 1 week off. May decrease the effectiveness of other medications, to prevent this take Marshmallow 1 hour after your other medications.

CROHN'S DISEASE

Other Herbs To Try: Wormwood, Boswellia, Turmeric, Marshmallow Root, Slippery Elm, Milk Thistle, Ginger Root, Licorice Root, Skullcap, Chicory Root, Cloves, Bromelain, L-Gutamine, Bentonite Clay, Vitamin D3, Fish Oil, Vitamin B12 , Cannabidiol (CBD), Qing Dai

Wormwood

- ✦ **Other Names:** Artemisia absinthium
- ✦ **Use:** Crohn's, Colitis, IBD/IBS, Sibo, Eliminates Intestinal Worms, Lowers Fever, Liver, Gallbladder, Migraines, Anorexia, Insomnia, Stomaches, Maleria, Treats E-coli, Pain, Flu
- ✦ **How to Take:** Tincture, Tea
- ✦ **Warnings:** Not meant for long term use!! Only take for 1 month each day then take 1 month off. High dose could cause nausea, vomiting, kidney issues. Not Recommended if Pregnant/Nursing, Allergic to Ragweed, if you have epilepsy or taking an anticonvulsant, or kidney disorders. Do not take if on warfain.

Boswellia

- ✦ **Other Names:** Boswellia serrata
- ✦ **Use:** Anti-Inflammatory, Crohn's, Colitis, IBD/IBS, Gout, Arthritis, Low back pain, Diarrhea, Fibromyalgia, Ringworm, Eases Digestion, Cramping, Pain, Anti-Fungal, Lowers Cholesterol, Protects Liver, Myositis, Repairs Blood Vessels
- ✦ **How to Take:** Capsule, Tablet
- ✦ **Warnings:** Can stimulate blood flow to uterus causing heavier period flow, may induce miscarriage in pregnant women. Could cause nausea, acid reflux, diarrhea, skin rashes when taking high doses.

-D-

<u>DEMENTIA</u> (See Alzheimers)

<u>DEPRESSION</u> (See Anxiety)

<u>DIABETES</u>

Other Herbs To Try: Cardamom, Chicory Root, Holy Basil, Kratom, Berberine, Garam masala, Milk Thistle, Cinnamon

Cardamom
- ✦ **Other Names:** Cardamum, Cardamom disambiguation
- ✦ **Use:** Diabetes Treatment, Treats Cavities, Cancer, Lowers Blood Pressures, Stomaches, Ulcers, Asthma
- ✦ **How to Take:** Capsule
- ✦ **Warnings:** N/A

Chicory Root
- ✦ **Other Names:** Cichorium Intybus
- ✦ **Use:** Manages Diabetes, Reduces Stress, Anti-Inflammatory, Liver, Manages Osteoarthritis, Aids Gut Health, Relives Constipation, Eczema, Regulates Thyroid, Treats IBD/IBS, Relives Bloating & Gas
- ✦ **How to Take:** Capsule, Tablet
- ✦ **Warnings:** Not recommended if Pregnant/Nursing. Some people allergic will have hives, rashes, itching, swelling.

-E-

ECZEMA
Other Herbs To Try: Licorice Root, Borage, Burdock Root, Witch Hazel, Fish Oil, Vitamin D3, Vitamin E

Licorice Root
- **Other Names:** Gycyrrhiza glabra
- **Use:** Fights Inflammation, Viral & Bacterial Infection, Eczema, Cleanses Colon, Reduces Muscle Spasms, Allergies, Asthma, Chronic Fatigue Syndrome, Depression, IBD/IBS, Menopause, Upper Respiratory Infection, Anti-Cancer properties
- **How to Take:** Capsule, Tablet
- **Warnings:** Not Recommended if Pregnant/Nursing or if you have diabetes, Glaucoma, heart disease, high blood pressure, history of stroke, severe menstrual problems. Not recommended for long term use!

Borage
- **Other Names:** Borago officinalis
- **Use:** Treats skin flare-ups, Eczema, Anti-Inflammatory, PMS, ADHD, Dermatitis, Menopause, Hormonal Imbalances, Chronic Fatigue Syndrome, Rheumatoid Arthritis, Stress, Diabetes, Colds, Cough, Fever, Pain, Preventing heart disease & stoke
- **How to Take:** Capsule, Tablet
- **Warnings:** Could case in some individuals Bloating, Soft Stools, Diarrhea, Blenching. Not recommend if Pregnant/Nursing, Not advised if you are taking warfarin as Borage thins the blood, Can interact with certain seizure medications Talk to your Dr. before taking.

ERECTILE DISFUNCTION

Other Herbs To Try: Horney Goat Weed

Horney Goat Weed

- **Other Names:** epimedium ,Yin-Yang-Huo, Herba Epimdii, Fairy Wings, Rowdy Lamb Herb, Barrenwort, Bishop's Hat, Icariin
- **Use:** Natural Aphrodisiac, Impotence, Increase testosterone , increases estrogen, Menopause, Improves Libido, Boosts Circulation, Vaginal Dryness, Normalized Cortisol Levels, Increase muscle mass, Prevents bone loss
- **How to Take:** Capsule, Extract
- **Warnings:** Possible side effects in some individuals increased thirst, dizziness, nauseas, nosebleeds. Can interfere with blood clotting, if you are currently taking meds for cancer, heart, liver or kidney disease consult your doctor.

EPILEPSY

Other Herbs To Try: Skullcap, Moringa, Kava, Bupleurum

Skullcap

- **Other Names:** Scutellaria laterfolia
- **Use:** Fights Cancer, Aids in sleep, Improves circulation, Strengthens heart muscle, Relieves muscle spasms, Cramps, Pain, Stress, Anxiety, Fatigue, Headache, Hyperactivity, Nervous Disorders, Rheumatism.
- **How to Take:** Capsule, Tablet
- **Warnings:** Should not be given to Children under 6.

-F-

FEVER
Other Herbs To Try: Goto Kola, Borage

Goto Kola
- ✦ **Other Names:** Centella asiatica
- ✦ **Use:** Reduces Fever, Eliminates excess fluids, Decreases Fatigue & Depression, Increases Sex Drive, Promotes Wound Healing, Varicose Veins, Kidney Stones, Poor appetite, Sleep disorders
- ✦ **How to Take:** Capsule, Tablet
- ✦ **Warnings:** May cause dermatitis if applied topically

FIBROMYALGIA
Other Herbs To Try: Holy Basil, Ashwagandha, Turmeric, D-Ribose, Magnesium Citrate, Vitamin D3, Fish Oil

D-Ribose
- ✦ **Other Names:** N/A
- ✦ **Use:** Fibromyalgia, Chronic Fatigue Syndrome, Heart Disease, Improves sleep, Increases Energy Levels, Sense of Well being, Decreases pain, Lowers Blood Sugar
- ✦ **How to Take:** Capsule, Tablet, Powder
- ✦ **Warnings:** Not Recommended if you take Insulin or other diabetic meds

<u>FLU</u> (See Common Cold)

<u>FREQUENT URINATION</u>
Other Herbs To Try: Saw Palmetto

Saw Palmetto
- ✦ **Other Names:** Serenoa repens
- ✦ **Use:** Acts as a Diuretic, Urinary Antiseptic, Reduces Frequent Urination (take at night), Stimulates Appetite, Inhibits production of dihydrotestosterone (testosterone), Prostate help, Improves Urinary tract in Men with benign prostatic hyperplasia, Enhances sexual function and sexual desire.
- ✦ **How to Take:** Capsule, Tablet
- ✦ **Warnings:** N/A

-G-

GALLBLADDER

Other Herbs To Try: Dandelion Root, Turmeric, Milk Thistle, Boldo, Devil's Claw

Dandelion Root
+ **Other Names:** Harpagophytum procumbens, Dandelion
+ **Use:** Acts as a Diuretic, Cleanses Blood & Liver, Cirrhosis of the Liver, Increases bile production, Improves Kidney Function, Pancreas, Spleen & Stomach, Relieves Menopause symptoms, Anemia, Boils, Breast Tumors, Constipation, Jaundice, Rheumatism, Breast Cancer
+ **How to Take:** Capsule, Tablet, Tea
+ **Warnings:** Not recommended to take with prescription diuretics, or persons with gallstones or biliary tract obstruction.

GOUT

Other Herbs To Try: Celery Seed Extract, Turmeric, Boswellia, Devil's Claw, Vitamin C, Mullein

Celery Seed
+ **Other Names:** Apium graveolens, Celery Seed Extract
+ **Use:** Gout, Arthritis, Reduces Blood Pressure, Relieves Muscle Spasms, Improves Appetite, Kidney Issues
+ **How to Take:** Capsule, Tablet
+ **Warnings:** Do Not take large amounts! Do Not eat seeds if you are pregnant!

GRAVE'S DISEASE (See Hyperthyroidism)

-H-

<u>HAY FEVER</u> (See Allergies)

<u>HEADACHE</u>
Other Herbs To Try: Turmeric, Feverfew, Butterbur

<u>HEART CONDITIONS</u>
Other Herbs To Try: Barberry, Skullcap, Berberine, Psyllium Husk

Barberry
- ✦ **Other Names:** Berberis vulgaris
- ✦ **Use:** Decreases Heart Rate, Slows Breathing, Reduces Bronchial Constriction, Kills Bacteria on Skin, Stimulates Intestinal Movement.
- ✦ **How to Take:** Capsule, Tablet
- ✦ **Warnings:** Do Not take if Pregnant/Nursing

HIVES/URTICARIA (See Allergies)

HYPERGLYCEMIA (High Blood Sugar)
Other Herbs To Try: Coriander, Ginseng, CoQ10

Coriander
✦ **Other Names:** Coriander Leaves, Coriander Seed
Chinese Parsley, Cilantro
✦ **Use:** Lowers Blood Sugar, Eases Digestive Discomfort,
Decreases Blood Pressure, Fights Food Poisoning,
Improves Cholesterol Levels, Improves Urinary Tract
Infections,Supports Healthy Menstrual Function,
Prevents Neurological Inflammation
✦ **How to Take:** Capsule, Tincture
✦ **Warnings:** Some individuals could experience sensitivity
to the sunlight, If you are allergic to aniseed, caraway, dill
weed, fennel or mugwort you could be allergic to
Coriander. Monitor your blood sugar levels closely if you
have diabetes.

<u>HYPERTENSION (High Blood Pressure)</u>

Other Herbs To Try: Asafoetida, Evening Primrose, Kratom, Linden,Barberry, Cardamom, Cat's Claw, Coriander

Asafoetida
- ✦ **Other Names:** Ferula asafoetida
- ✦ **Use:** Lowers Blood Pressure, Asthma Relief, Whopping Cough, Bronchitis, Helps treat IBS, Gas, Bloating, Cramping, Controls Blood Sugar, Reduces Flatulence
- ✦ **How to Take:** Capsule, Tincture
- ✦ **Warnings:** Taking more than suggested on bottle could cause upset stomach, diarrhea, and urination discomfort, Not recommended for Children, Pregnant/ Nursing Mothers. Do Not take if you have a bleeding disorder, epilepsy or taking blood thinners.

<u>HYPERTHYROIDISM (Over Active Thyroid)</u>

Other Herbs To Try: Bugleweed, Motherwort, Lemon Balm , L-carnitine

Bugelweed

✦ **Other Names:** Lycopus virginicus
✦ **Use:** Thyroid suppressant, Decreases symptoms of hyperthyroidism, Coughs, Calms heart palpitations, Treats fevers, Moderates estrogen levels
✦ **How to Take:** Capsule
✦ **Warnings:** Could cause Hives, Tingling in mouth, Headaches, Abdominal pain. Not recommended if Pregnant/Nursing, Be careful if Diabetic as it will lower blood sugar levels, Not recommended if going though chemotherapy, or if taking Thyroid meds. If you have a scheduled surgery discontinue use 2 week prior.

Motherwort

✦ **Other Names:** Leonurus cardiaca
✦ **Use:** Thyroid, Menstrual disorders, Menopausal Symptoms, Rheumatic Problems, Headaches, Insomnia, Vertigo, Relieves Childbirth pain
✦ **How to Take:** Capsule
✦ **Warnings:** Not Recommended if Pregnant (until the onset of labor), Not recommended for persons with clotting disorders, high blood pressure, or heart disease

HYPOTHYROIDISM
(Under Active Thyroid)

Other Herbs To Try: Bayberry, Selenium, Holy Basil, Ashwagandha, L-Tyrosine, Iodine, L-Glutamine

Bayberry
- ✦ **Other Names:** Myrica cerifera
- ✦ **Use:** Stimulates Thyroid, Decongestant, Aids in Circulation, Reduces Fever, Ulcers, Good for eyes, Boosts Immune System
- ✦ **How to Take:** Capsule
- ✦ **Warnings:** Should Not be used at high dosages or for prolonged periods. May irritate sensitive stomaches

Selenium
- ✦ **Other Names:** N/A
- ✦ **Use:** Regulates Thyroid, Fights aging process, Boosts Immune System, Cancer, Improves Blood Flow, Reduces Asthma Symptoms, Boosts Fertility
- ✦ **How to Take:** Capsule
- ✦ **Warnings:** Not recommended to take high doses without consulting Doctor first. May interact with other meds such as antacids, chemotherapy drugs, corticosteroids, niacin, cholesterol lowering meds & birth control pills.

-I-

IMMUNE SYSTEM (Boost)

Other Herbs To Try: Arrow Root, Astragalus, Elderberry, Zinc, Holy Basil, Black Currant, Cat's Claw

Arrowroot

✦ **Other Names:** Maranta arundinacea, Zamia integrifolia, Manihot esculenta, Kudzu, Pueraria lobata
✦ **Use:** Anti-Inflammatory, Boosts Immune System, Reduces Diarrhea & Constipation, Treats Urinary Tract Infections, Relieves gums and soreness in mouth, IBS
✦ **How to Take:** Capsule, Tea
✦ **Warnings:** N/A

IMPOTENCE (See Erectile Disfunction)

<u>INDIGESTION (Heart Burn)</u>

Other Herbs To Try: L-Glutamine, Bromelain, Magnesium

L-Glutamine
✦ **Other Names:** N/A
✦ **Use:** Calms acid reflux, Relaxes stomach, Improves Gastrointestinal health, Boosts Immune System, Weight loss, Helps fight off infection, Crohn's, Colitis, IBD/IBS, Ulcers, Boosts Brain Health, Diarrhea, Helpful for Hypothyroidism, Promotes Muscle Growth, Improves Diabetes
✦ **How to Take:** Capsule, Tea
✦ **Warnings:** N/A

<u>INSOMNIA</u>

Other Herbs To Try: Valerian Root, Kava, Chamomile, Lemon Balm, Skullcap, Gaba

Valerian Root
- ✦ **Other Names:** Valerian, Valeriana officinalis
- ✦ **Use:** Sedative, Insomnia, Promotes Better Sleep, Longer Sleep Periods, Improves Circulation, Reduces Mucus from Colds, Anxiety, High Blood Pressure, IBS, Menstrual & Muscle Cramps, Nervousness, Pain, Stress, Ulcers
- ✦ **How to Take:** Capsule, Tincture
- ✦ **Warnings:** N/A

Kava
- ✦ **Other Names:** Kava Kava, Kava Root, Piper methysticum
- ✦ **Use:** Mental Relaxation, Physical Relaxation, Insomnia, Diuretic, Relieves Gastrointestinal issues, Relieves Muscle Spasms, Eases Pain, Anxiety, Menopausal Symptoms, Urinary Tract Infections, Anti-convulsive, Protects Nervous System
- ✦ **How to Take:** Capsule
- ✦ **Warnings:** Causes Drowsiness, Usually works within 2 hours of taking it (don't operate heavy machinery or drive after taking). Should Not be combined with Alcohol, Not Recommenced for Persons under the age of 18, or if Pregnant/Nursing. Not Recommend if taking meds for depression (anti-anxiety drugs), of if you have liver of skin diseases. Beware that large amounts for extended periods of time may worsen liver function.

<u>IRON DEFICIENCY</u> (See Anemia)

<u>IRRITABLE BOWL DISEASE</u>
(See Crohn's Disease)

<u>IRRITABLE BOWEL SYNDROME</u>
(See Crohn's Disease)

-K-

<u>KIDNEY STONES</u>
(See Gallbladder)
Other Herbs to try: Dandelion Root, Psyllium Husk

-L-

<u>LARYNGITIS</u> (See Cough)

<u>LIVER DISEASE</u>
Other Herbs To Try: Boldo, Buplerum

Boldo
- ✦ **Other Names:** Peumus boldus
- ✦ **Use:** Liver Tonic, Liver ailments, Diuretic, Laxative, Antibiotic, Anti-Inflammatory, Excretes Uric Acid, Stimulates Digestion, Gallstones
- ✦ **How to Take:** Capsule
- ✦ **Warnings:** N/A

<u>LUNG DISEASE</u> (See Asthma/Cough)

LUPUS
Other Herbs To Try: Bromelian, Turmeric, Ginger, Holy Basil, Buplerum

Bromelian
✦ **Other Names:** N/A
✦ **Use:** Anti-Inflammatory, Prevents blood clots, Edema, Reduces Swelling, Soothes & Relaxes tense & Inflamed muscles & connective tissues, ACL Tears, Sprained Ankles, Tendonitis, Allergies, Arthritis, Joint Pain, Heart Burn, Diarrhea, Autoimmune disorders, Cancer, IBD/IBS, Crohn's, Colitis, Sinus Infections, Bronchitis, Sinusitis, Speeds up recovery after surgery
✦ **How to Take:** Capsule, Tea
✦ **Warnings:** Prevents Blood clotting, Be careful if on blood thinning meds, Avoid taking before surgery

LYME DISEASE
Other Herbs To Try: Devil's Claw, Astragalus Root, Cat's Claw

Devi's Claw
✦ **Other Names:** Harpagophytum procumbens, Grapple Plant, Wood Spider
✦ **Use:** Lyme Disease, Relives Pain, Reduces Inflammation, Back Pain, Arthritis, Digestive Stimulant, Diuretic, Sedative, Rheumatism, Diabetes, Allergies, Liver, Gallbladder, Kidney disorders, Gout, Menopausal Symptoms, Migraines
✦ **How to Take:** Capsule
✦ **Warnings:** Not Recommended if Pregnant/Nursing, Some people may experience Gastrointestinal problems.

-M-

MENIERE'S DISEASE

Other Herbs To Try: Butcher's Broom, Dandelion Root, Echinacea, Gingko Biloba, Ginseng, Lipase Enzymes

Butcher's Broom
- ✦ **Other Names:** Ruscus aculeatus
- ✦ **Use:** Treats Meniere's Disease, Reduces Inflammation, Carpal Tunnel, Circulatory Disorders, Edema, Raynaud's Phenomenon, Thrombophlebitis, Varicose Veins, Vertigo, Good for Bladder & Kidneys
- ✦ **How to Take:** Capsule
- ✦ **Warnings:** Note: Take with Vitamin C for best results

MENOPAUSE

Other Herbs To Try: Chaste Tree, Black Cohosh, Dandelion Root, Evening Primrose, Mugwort, Dong quai

Chaste Tree

✦ **Other Names:** Vitex agnus-castus, Chasteberry, Vitex
✦ **Use:** Normalizes Hormonal Levels, Regulates Hormones, Regulates Menstrual Cycle, Calming, Soothing, Relieves Muscle Cramps, PMS
✦ **How to Take:** Capsule
✦ **Warnings:** Not Recommended if Pregnant/Nursing, Not Recommended for Children

Black Cohosh

✦ **Other Names:** Cimicifuga racemosa, Snakeroot
✦ **Use:** Relieves Menopausal Symptoms, Lowers Blood Pressure & Cholesterol Levels, Menstrual Cramps, Back Pain, Morning Sickness, Pain, Induces Labor, Poisonous Snake Bites, Arthritis
✦ **How to Take:** Capsule
✦ **Warnings:** Not Recommended if Pregnant (to induce Labor take small amount 2 weeks before due date), Long Term use could cause Liver problems.

<u>MENSTRUAL CRAMPS</u>

Other Herbs To Try: Evening Primrose, Ginger Root

Evening Primrose
- ✦ **Other Names:** Oenothera biennis, Primrose
- ✦ **Use:** Natural Estrogen Promoter, Treats Menstrual Cramps & Heavy Bleeding, Hot Flashes, Aids in Weight Loss, Reduces High Blood Pressure, Treats Alcoholism
- ✦ **How to Take:** Capsule
- ✦ **Warnings:** Not Recommend if Pregnant/Nursing, Best if taken the week before your cycle and during, then take break from it.

<u>MIGRAINE</u>

Other Herbs To Try: Feverfew, Butterbur, Chaste Tree, Kava, Devil's Claw, Magnesium

Feverfew
- ✦ **Other Names:** Chrysanthemum parthenium ,Featherfew, Featherfoil
- ✦ **Use:** Headaches, Migraines, Menstrual Issues, Muscle Tension, Pain, Muscle Spasms, Increases Bronchial Tube Mucus, Stimulates Appetite, Stimulates Urine Contractions, Arthritis, Colitis, IBD
- ✦ **How to Take:** Capsule
- ✦ **Warnings:** Not Recommended if Pregnant/Nursing, Be careful if taking blood thinning meds as Feverfew will thin your blood, Do Not take over the counter painkillers when using Feverfew as the combination could result in internal bleeding

<u>MULTIPLE SCLEROSIS (MS)</u>

Other Herbs To Try: Cinnamon, Evening Primrose, Turmeric, Ginger, CoQ10

Cinnamon
- ✦ **Other Names:** Cinnamomum verum
- ✦ **Use:** Relieves MS Symptoms, Diarrhea, Nausea, Congestion, Enhances Digestion, Fights Fungal Infection, Diabetes, Weight Loss, Yeast Infections
- ✦ **How to Take:** Capsule
- ✦ **Warnings:** Not Recommended to use in large amounts when Pregnant

-P-

PAIN

Other Herbs To Try: Turmeric, Kratom, Willow Bark, Poppy Seed, Kava, Noni, Cannabidiol (CBD)

Turmeric
✦ **Other Names:** Curcuma longa
✦ **Use:** Anti-Inflammatory, Pain Relief, Liver, Aids in Circulation, Headache, Bursitis, Lowers Cholesterol, Improves blood vessels, Antibiotic, Anticancer, Arthritis, Psoriasis, Alzheimer's disease, IBD/IBS, Crohn's, Colitis
✦ **How to Take:** Capsule, Tincture, Tea
✦ **Warnings:** Extended use could result in stomach issues, Not Recommenced for persons with biliary tract obstruction

Kratom
✦ **Other Names:** Mitragyna speciosa, Bali, Maeng Da, Red Vein Thai, Red Vein Kali, Green Vein Kali
✦ **Use:** Anti-Inflammatory, Pain Relief, Increases Energy, PTSD Symptoms, Opiate Withdrawal Relief, Enhances Mood, Anxiety, Depression, Stimulates Immune System, Lowers Blood Sugar, Enhances Sexual Function
✦ **How to Take:** Capsule, Tea
✦ **Warnings:** May cause constipation, digestive and liver issues with extended use, Not Recommend if Pregnant/ Nursing

PNEUMONIA (See Cough)

POST TRAUMATIC STRESS DISORDER (PTSD) (See Anxiety, Pain)

Other Herbs To Try: Buplerum, Ginkgo Biloba, Kava, St. John's Wort, Kratom

POSTNATAL DEPRESSION (See Anxiety)

PROSTATE (See Frequent Urination)

PSORIASIS (See Eczema)

-R-

RHEUMATOID ARTHRITIS (See Arthritis)

-S-

SHINGLES

Other Herbs To Try: Echinacea, Zinc, Vitamin B12

Echinacea
- ✦ **Other Names:** Echinacea species
- ✦ **Use:** Anti-Inflammatory, Fights off Bacterial/Viruses, Boosts Immune System, Shingle Relief, Colds, Flu, Infections, Stimulates White Blood Cells
- ✦ **How to Take:** Capsule, Tinctures
- ✦ **Warnings:** Do Not take for longer than 3 weeks. Not to be used if allergic to Ragwood.

SIBO (See Crohn's)

SINUSITIS

Other Herbs To Try: Horehound, Elderberry, Bromelian, Horseradish Root

Horehound
- ✦ **Other Names:** Marrubium vulgare
- ✦ **Use:** Sinusitis Relief, Decreases thick mucus, Sinus Infection, Bronchitis, Boosts Immune System, Indigestion, Loss of Appetite, Bloating, Hay Fever, Respiratory issues
- ✦ **How to Take:** Capsule
- ✦ **Warnings:** Large doses could cause irregular heart beat

<u>SORE THROAT</u> (See Cough)

<u>STOMACHACHE/ABDOMINAL PAIN</u>
Other Herbs To Try: Clove, Ginger, Milk Thistle

Clove
+ **Other Names:** Syzgium aromaticum
+ **Use:** Relieves Digestive Issues, Calms Stomachache, Toothache, Mouth Pain, Antiseptic
+ **How to Take:** Capsule, Tincture
+ **Warnings:** Clove Oil is very strong use with caution, can cause irritation in some individuals in large doses

STRESS (See Anxiety)

STROKE (Prevention & Post Stroke)

Other Herbs To Try: Citicoline, Borage, Ashwagandha, Ginseng, Ginseng Biloba

Citicoline
✦ **Other Names:** N/A
✦ **Use:** Helps Retain Memory, Good for Memory Loss, Cognitive Decline, Liver, Nerve Functions, Muscle Movement, Boosts Energy Levels, Supports Central Nervous System, Supports Healthy Pregnancy
✦ **How to Take:** Capsule
✦ **Warnings:** Take Recommend dose or you could experience symptoms such as diarrhea, nauseas, high blood pressure

-T-

THYROID (See Hyper/Hypo-Thyroidisum)

TUBERCULOSIS (TB)
Other Herbs To Try: Rhodiola rosea, Astragalus

TUMOR (See Cancer)
Other Herbs To Try: Dandelion Root, Astragulaus, Galangal

-U-

<u>ULCERATIVE COLITIS</u> (See Crohn's Disease)

<u>URINARY TRACT INFECTION (UTI)</u>

Other Herbs To Try: Arrowroot, Birch, D-Mannose, Garlic, Cranberry, Clove

Arrowroot
- ✦ **Other Names:** Maranta arundinacea, Zamia integrifolia, Florida Arrowroot
- ✦ **Use:** Anti-Inflammatory, Treats and Prevents UTI's, Digestive Aid, Boosts Immune System, Treats Diarrhea, Reduces Abdominal Pain
- ✦ **How to Take:** Capsule, Tea, Tincture
- ✦ **Warnings:** N/A

-V-

<u>VERTIGO</u> (See Meniere's Disease)
Other Herbs To Try:Ginkgo Biloba, Ginger

<u>VIRUS</u> (See Common Cold)

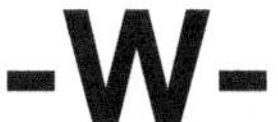

-W-

WEIGHT LOSS

Other Herbs To Try: Cayenne, Black Currant, Ginseng, Saffron, L-Glutamine, Ginger

Cayenne
- ✦ **Other Names:** Capsicum frutescens, C. annum, Capsicum, Hot Pepper, Red Pepper
- ✦ **Use:** Aids in Weight Loss, Aids in Digestion, Improves Circulation, Stops Bleeding Ulcers, Heart, Kidneys, Lung, Spleen, Pancreas, Arthritis, Wards off Colds, Sinus Infection, Sore Throats
- ✦ **How to Take:** Capsule
- ✦ **Warnings:** Avoid Contact with Eyes

WHOPPING COUGH (See Cough)

Other Herbs To Try: Ginger, Turmeric, Licorice Root

Ailments List-Herbs

- **ADHD:** Gaba, Rhodiola rosea, Fish Oil, B-Complex (B6 Vitamins), phosphatidylserine, Kava, Ginkgo Biloba
- **Allergies:** Stinging nettle, Butterbur, Garlic, Rosemary, Turmeric
- **Alzheimer's :** Butterbur, Ginkgo biloba 120 mg day, Phosphatidylserine 300 mg day, Ginseng, CoQ10, Vitamin D3, Fish Oil, Rosemary Essential oil , Berberine, Ashwagandha
- **Anemia:** Moringa
- **Anxiety:** Gaba, Ashwagandha (adaptogen), Kava Root, Vitamin B Complex, Magnesium, Kratom, Holy Basil, Skullcap, Buplerum, Chamomile
- **Arthritis:** Stinging nettle, Ginger, Turmeric, Boswellia, Glucosamine, MSM, Fish Oil, Evening Primrose, Noni, Holy Basil,   Vitamin B6, Skullcap, Borage, Cat's claw, Bromelain
- **Asthma:** Ginseng, Astragalus, Butterbur, Vitamin D, Magnesium, Echinacea
- **Autism**: Poria Cocos, Panax ginseng, Acorus gramineus, Schisandra chinensis, Glycyrrhiza uralensis
- **Bacteria Infection:** Berberine
- **Bipolar disorder:** Holy Basil, Ashwagandha, Ginseng, Rhodiola, St. John's Wort, Fish Oil
- **Blood Pressure** (see hypertension)
- **Boost Memory:** (see Alzheminers)
- **Bursitis:** Turmeric, Glucosamine, Bromelian
- **Cancer:** Vitamin B12, Vitamin D3, Turmeric, Cordycep & Reishi Mushrooms, Soursop (gwanabana), Kava, Wormwood, Skullcap, Basil, Bay leaf, Black Currant, Boswellia, Cardmom, Cat's Claw, Thyme, Galangal, Ginger
- **Cholesterol (high) :** Turmeric, Garlic, Fish Oil, CoQ10, Hawthorne, Berberine, Ginger root, Milk Thistle, Thyme
- **Constipation:** Aloe Vera, Chia Seeds, Magnesium, Flaxseed oil, Psyllium Husk, Slippery Elm, Triphala
- **Common Cold:** Elderberry, Ginger, Garlic, Echinacea, Zinc , Vitamin D, Oregano Oil (500 mg 2x day), Black Currant
- **Cough:** Ginger tea, Vitamin C, Zinc Lozenges, Honey, Licorice root, Elderberry, Mullein, Linden, Asafoetida, Marshmallow root, Slippery Elm
-

- **Crohn's disease:** Wormwood, Turmeric, Boswellia, Slippery Elm, Bentonite clay, Milk Thistle, Vitamin D3, Fish Oil, Vitamin B12, Ginger root, Licorice root, Marshmallow Root, L-Gutamine Powder , Skullcap, Chicory root, Bromelain, Cannabidiol (CBD), Clove, Qing Dai
- **Dementia:** (see Alzheimers)
- **Depression**: (see Anxiety)
- **Diabetes:** Kratom, Holy Basil, Barberry, Berberine, Burdock root, Cardamom, Chicory Root, Garam Masala, Milk Thistle, Cinnamon
- **Eczema :** Licorice root, Vitamin D3, Vitamin E, Witch Hazel, Fish Oil, Borage, Burdock root
- **Erectile disfunction:** Horney Goat Weed
- **Epilepsy:** Kava, Skullcap, Bupleurum, Moringa
- **Fever:** Borage, Gotu Kola
- **Fibromyalgia:** Holy Basil, Ashwagandha, Turmeric, D-Ribose, Vitamin D3, Fish Oil, Magnesium Citrate
- **Flu** (see common cold)
- **Frequent Urination (at night):** Saw palmetto
- **Gallbladder :** Turmeric, Milk Thistle, Dandelion Root, Bolda , Devil's Claw, Psyllium Husk
- **Gout:** Celery seed extract**,** Turmeric, Boswellia, Devil's Claw Vitamin C, Mullein
- **Graves' disease:** (See Hyperthyroidism)
- **Hay fever** (see allergies)
- **Heart conditions:** Skullcap, Barberry, Berberine, Psyllium Husk
- **Headache:** Feverfew, Willow bark, Kava
- **Hives/Urticaria:** (see allergies)
- **Hyperglycemia (high blood sugar):** Coriander seed, Ginseng, CoQ10
- **Hypertension (high blood pressure):** Evening Primrose, Kratom, Linden, Asafoetida, Barberry, Cardamom, Cat's Claw, Coriander seed
- **Hyperthyroidism (Over active thyroid) :** Bugleweed, Motherwort, Lemon Balm
- **Hypothyroidism (under active thyroid):** Holy Basil, Ashwagandha, Selenium, Iodine, L-Tyrosine, Bayberry
- **Immune System (boost):** Astragalus, Elderberry, Zinc, Holy Basil, Arrowroot, Black Currant , Cat's Claw
- **Impotence (see Erectile disfunction)**

- **Indigestion (Heart Burn)** L-Glutamine, Magnesium, Bromelain
- **Insomnia:** Gaba, skullcap, Kava, Lemon Balm, Chamomile, Valerian root
- **Iron deficiency** (see anemia)
- **Irritable Bowl Disease (IBD)** (see Crohn's)
- **Irritable Bowel Syndrome (IBS)** (see Crohn's)
- **Kidney stones:** Dandelion root, Psyllium Husk (see Gallbladder)
- **Laryngitis :** (see cough)
- **Liver disease:** Boldo, Buplerum
- **Lung disease** (see pneumonia, asthma, tuberculosis)
- **Lupus:** Turmeric, Ginger, Holy Basil, Buplerum, Bromelian
- **Lyme disease :** Astragalus root, Buckthorn bark, Cat's Claw, Devils Claw
- **Meniere's Disease :** Dandelion Root, Echinacea, Ginkgo Biloba, Ginseng, Lipase Enzyme, Noni, Butcher's broom
- **Menopause:** Dandelion Root, Evening Primrose, Chaste Tree, Black Cohosh, Mugwort, Dong quai
- **Menstrual cramps:** Evening Primrose, Ginger root,
- **Migraine:** Butterbur, Chaste tree, Feverfew, Kava, Devil's Claw, Magnesium
- **Multiple sclerosis (MS) :** Evening Primrose, Turmeric, Cinnamon, Ginger, CoQ10
- **Pain:** Kratom, Turmeric, Willow bark, Poppy Seed, Kava, Noni, Cannabidiol (CBD)
- **Pneumonia:** Berberine (also see cough)
- **Post traumatic stress disorder (PTSD)** (See Pain/Anxiety) Chai Hu, Ginkgo biloba, Kava root, St. John's wort, Kratom
- **Postnatal depression:** (see anxiety)
- **Prostate:** (see frequent urination)
- **Psoriasis** (see eczema)
- **Rheumatoid arthritis** (see arthritis)
- **Shingles:** Echinacea, Zinc, Vitmin B12
- **SIBO (See Crohn's/Ulcerative Colitis)**
- **Sinusitis:** Horehound, Horseradish root, Bromelian, Elderberry
- **Sore throat** (see cough)
- **Stomachache/Abdominal pain:** Ginger, Milk Thistle, Clove
- **Stress:** (see Anxiety)
- **Stroke:** Borage, Ashwagandha, Ginseng, Citicoline, Ginkgo Biloba

- **Thyroid** (see hyper/hypo-thyroidism)
- **Tuberculosis (TB):** Rhodiola, Astragalus,
- **Tumors:** Dandelion root, Astragualus root, Galangal, (see Cancer)
- **Ulcerative Colitis** (see Crohn's)
- **Urinary tract infection (UTI) :** Arrowroot, D-Mannose, Garlic, Birch
- **Vertigo:** Ginkgo biloba, Ginger, (see Menieres Disease)
- **Virus (see cold)**
- **Weight loss:** Black Currant , Cayenne Pepper, Ginseng, Saffron, L-Glutamine, Ginger
- **Whooping cough:** (See Cough) Ginger, Turmeric, Licorice Root, Black Currant

Chapter 2

WELCOME TO THE

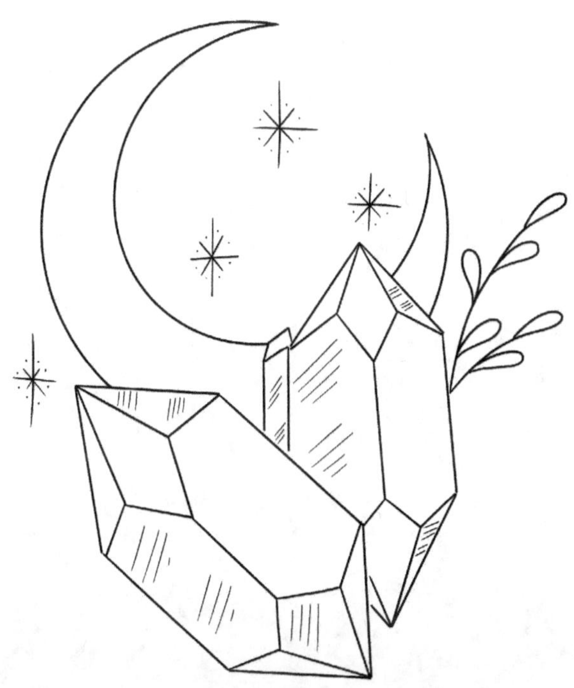

Mineral Kingdom

SECTION 1
CRYSTAL HISTORY

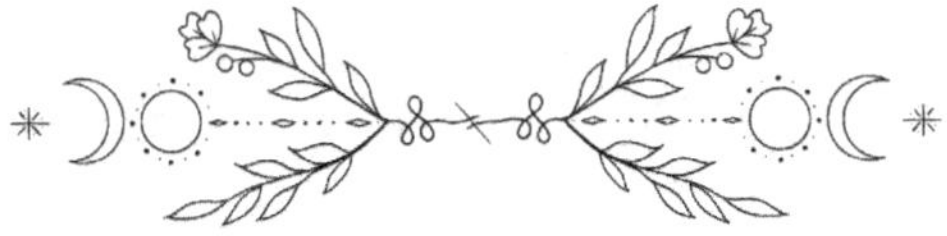

Crystals being used for healing purposes has been around since the beginning of man. It spans many centuries and has been part of some religions as well.

In ancient Egypt, they found in the tombs information about Crystals used for healing as well as in ancient religious texts from all around the world!

It starts all the way back … as early as 4000 BCE. The most earliest documentations come from this time period. These documents were from the ancient Sumerians in Mesopotamia.

Our ancient Sumerian ancestors enjoyed working with Crystals made of Hematite and Gypsum (Selenite) to create cylinder seals that they then would inscribe their images and phrases in cuneiform.

It was also their form of a diary. Including information such as events, births, marriages, and religious ceremonies.

Hematite and Selenite are both known for their protective properties, therefore these cylinders usually were kept in the temples and taken out and used during spiritual ceremonies.

The most well known set of ancients who worked with Crystals was the Egyptians.

Individuals who were of royalty, or in a high social ranking would adorn themselves with different Crystals. Some of the most favorite Crystal of Ancient Egypt was Lapis Lazuli.

Lapis Lazuli was found in jewelry pieces along side other Crystals such as Carnelian, Turquoise, and Calcite. They also enjoyed Gold.

King Tut's mask was made of Gold and Lapis Lazuli . What they did was they crushed up Lapis Lazuli, and used it to paint around King Tut's eyes and eyebrows. Pretty much anywhere you see the deep dark blue color is Lapis Lazuli.

The Egyptian's considered Lapis Lazuli to be associated with the Goddess Isis, the Goddess of the sky. So it makes sense why they used it in King Tut's mask, as his Spirit transitioned to the non-physical.

Even now, Lapis Lazuli is a treasured piece that people still enjoy to work with and wear! It's amazing qualities range from increasing your intuition, enhancing your communication skills, and brings about protection.

It has also been found that the Ancient Egyptians were buried with Quartz Crystals on their foreheads, allowing safe travels to the Spirit world.

Being the most popular Crystal in the Egyptian time… the women would crush up Lapis Lazuli and use it as make up! Now… let me just say, I don't recommend trying this at home! But, they used what they had back then.

Ancient Greece where also known to work with Crystals.
In greek the word they called Crystals was Krustallos which translates into ice. The Ancient Greeks believe that Clear Quartz Crystals were etheric ice sent down from the heavens.

Our Crystal called Amethyst, is derived by the Ancient Greeks.
It translates to "not to intoxicate."
The myth was that God Dionysus aka Bacchus (the god of wine) was inebriated and Goddess Diana worked with Amethyst to help sober him up.

Todays use with Amethyst still holds true, as it's known for it's ability to remove addiction and also helps you become sober, just as it did many centuries ago!

As we move forward in the years we hit the middle ages, where practicing the use of Crystal healing really started to shine!

In 300 CE to 1500 CE more research was being done on the healing abilities of Crystals. They started to learn that Crystals had a metaphysical tie as well as a physical one. Allowing them to work with Crystals for their Spiritual properties as well as healing.

In the middle ages Christianity was on the rise, and thus discouraged some of the ancient practices of working with healing Crystals.

Moving onward to the 20th century, working with Crystals started to decline. By the early 1900's it was not something practiced as much as in times of old.

However… as time progressed and we make it to the 1970's-1980's, this was when the use of Crystals for healing purposes were having a rebirth! During this time, Crystal therapy started to emerge as a meaning of healing the physical body, mind, emotions and spirit.

These practices are still being exercised to this day!

It's pretty exciting to see how long Crystals have been there supporting and helping us along the way. Crystals have been there for hundreds of years to bring us protection and peace.

These amazing Crystal beings are ready and willing to assist us, but they will only assist people who have fully opened themselves up to their loving powerful healing gifts.

We must always be grateful for their sacrifice and love.

As you carry onward in this section, keep in mind you will notice me using the term Mineral and Crystal interchangeability . They are in fact one in the same, just to avoid any confusion.

~ "Heal Yourself Holistically" ~ Bridget M. Shoup ~

SECTION 2
HOW CRYSTALS WORK

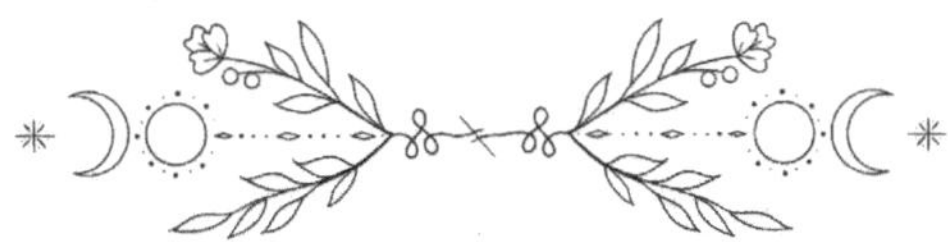

The Formation Of Crystals

Crystals have been around well... as long as the Earth has been! They are found deep within the layer of Gaia, our Mother Earth!

The Earth began as this whirling cloud of gas, that contracted into a hot molten ball.

Over eons, thin laters of this molten material called magma cooled into the crust of the Earth. It continues to boil, and new Crystals are found as time has progressed forward!

Superheated, these lovely little Crystal friends rise towards the surface over time. The stress and movement of the Earth causes these Crystals to show themselves to us!

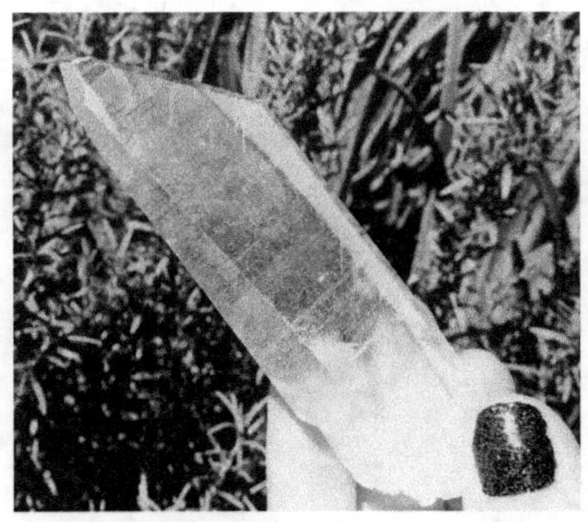

There are a few methods as to how Crystals develop.

Some Crystals take their time, and for them... development is a slow process!
While others grow in gas bubbles, as they form into the larger Crystals that we see today!

Then there are some Crystals who are ready to get on with life and take the fastest approach to growth! During this process the Crystal won't grow to be as large, but is still just as powerful in it's energetic properties!

Sometimes Crystals can't make up their mind! They will start to grow, and they get interrupted and that is when we get the cool phantom Crystals or self healed Crystals you see today.

Crystals go by many names! Some of the names you will hear them being referred to is Minerals, Gems, or Stones. Either way, they are one in the same!

There are more than 4,000 different types of Minerals in the Mineral Kingdom, with new ones found each day! !! That's a lot of Crystal Friends to explore!

Just like us, no two Crystals are alike!

What is a Crystal?

A Crystal is a Mineral with a regularly repeating internal molecule structure.   Also known as a Crystalline lattice that forms from building block like units of matter.

Crystals are the Earths DNA!!

A chemical imprint for evolution. Some of these Crystal friends have been subjected to enormous pressure within Gaia, while others grew in chambers deep underground.

As that was true from some of our Crystal friends, others had a different up bringing. Some were formed in layers, while others dripped into being.

This perfect molecule structure is what makes a Crystal a Crystal!
They are made up of amazing geometric shapes, connected to sacred geometry. With this stability they are born to assist us, allowing us to find stability within ourselves.
They share their focus and high vibrational energy with us.

Crystals are able to absorb, conserve, focus and emit energy!
How cool is that!?
The ability to stay in that high vibrational state is a consistent one with a Crystal. You see Crystals are not like us humans in that way!

The Crystals entrain with our energy, allowing us to mimic their high vibration… or what I like to call the "syncing up" process!

It's like when you get in your car and your bluetooth system needs to sync up with your phone, well that's what we do with Crystals! As we continue to work with them, they start to bring balance and stability to us! We will start to vibrate higher and take on their stability as our own.

Crystals each have their own list of amazing abilities to assist us.
They are like prescriptions really, they each have a special way to help us! Each Crystal is different, and they aid us in achieving a better way of life! It's neat to know they can assist us within all our bodies (emotional, mental, physical, spiritual).

Humans vs Crystals

Humans are made of 60% water!
Crystals are made up of practically none!

Due to this fact, us Humans come out of balance from time to time! We have to work at keeping our energy and emotions more consistently in a high vibrational state.

Whereas Crystals, are made with that perfection and stability from the beginning, allowing them to stay in that constant high vibration!

One thing we have in common with Crystals, is that we humans are made up of Crystals too. Did you know that your teeth and bones are made of a Crystal? Yep, it's called Hydroxyapatite $(Ca5(PO4)3(OH)$.

Another thing we have in common is, we both have Souls!

I believe that each Crystal has a Soul. I like to call them Crystal Devas!! Other names some people call them is Crystal Beings, or Oversouls. The reason why I like the name Crystal Deva, is that in Sanskrit Deva translates into "Shining One" and they most certainly are!

It's very important to recognize the Crystal Deva's and thank them for their assistance. They agreed to come here and be torn from their roots, deep down within Gaia. They have offered themselves up selflessly to assist us on our journey.

As they are here with a mission to serve, it's still imperative that we acknowledge this and give thanks.

I personally thank them verbally all the time. Another thing I like to do, is physically kiss them.

Also keep in mind, as our Crystal friends help us by removing discomfort... and send their love and healing in it's place... the low vibrational stuff (pain, sadness, hurt, fear) has to go somewhere!

Good Crystal hygiene is a must! Let's learn how.

Crystal Care

Crystals are like buckets and can only hold so much energy before they are full up and can no longer assist you! Once you "empty the bucket" (cleansing) then they can continue to assist you. This is especially important if you worked with a Crystal to remove pain from your body! The Crystal takes it on! So, it's important to make it a ritual to remove these lower vibrations from your Crystals from time to time.

You would want to smudge your Crystals, a way to cleansing them for the following reasons: You got a new Crystal, Someone touched it, You worked with it to remove pain/emotions from yourself.

Cleansing Methods:

1. Sage
2. Palo Santo
3. Water
4. Sound

Not all Crystals can be cleansed in water, in fact…water could dissolve certain types of Crystals, for example… Selenite. Best and safest cleansing methods are Sage, Palo Santo or even Sound.

Smudging

The process is quite simple, all you do is light your Sage/Palo Santo and once it's smoking you pass your Crystal through the smoke and say something like:
" Please remove any low or negative vibrations from this Crystal."

Other methods to cleanse your Crystals is by Sound.
You can either place your Crystals near a Crystal Singing Bowl or ring a bell, or sound your tingshas. This process will break up any stale or un-useful energy within the Crystal.

If you don't properly cleanse your Crystals things can start to happen! They could break, crack, go missing, or just won't be of the best assistance for you anymore. So if you ever have any of these things happen to you… think back, when was the last time you cleansed your Crystal Friend?

Charging

The next step would be to allow them some ample recharge time!

Now that you have cleansed your Crystals, you have a few more steps to go to getting your Crystal in its highest vibration possible. Charging is the next step!!

Allowing your Crystals some charging time is very important as it not only gives these hard workers a much needed break, but it allows a full refreshing battery charge so to speak! This process will also allow them to continue to share their high vibration with you!

Charging Methods:
1. Sun
2. Moon

Sun and Moon are the best ways to charge your Crystals! The way I like to do this is place my Crystals on a plate and set them outside. My preferred method is Moonlight, for a few different reasons. For one, some Crystals are photosensitive (Jade, Amethyst, Fluorite, etc) and will fade with time with too much sun exposer. Second reason, some Crystals like Clear Quartz can actually start fires, as it refracts the light of the sun…so be careful!

When placing them under the Sunlight or Moonlight, you can leave them outside for at least 3 hours. When I do a Moon charge, I like to leave them out all night and collect them in the morning.

Gratitude

Last Step…Gratitude!
Make sure you thank your Crystal Friends for being apart of your life and always assisting you!

I personally like to kiss my Crystals too, just showing extra love and affection for them always supporting me!

How To Work With Crystals

O Carry Them On You:

There are a few ways you can begin to work with your Crystals!
The easiest way to start to entrain with them is by having them on
you! This means carry them with you!! In your pocket, your bra
(that's my method of carry), purse or pouch.

Here is something I tell my Clients when they start working with
Crystals! Crystals are like Wifi….they will only help you when you're
near them. So think of the Crystal like the Wifi Signal. When you're
at home, and the Crystal is with you at home…. that energy exchange
between you is happening.

However say you have to go to work. If you leave your Crystal at
home, as you begin to drive away the signal gets weaker and weaker
until the signal is completely lost!
(((the only exception to this is if you have a Crystal Grid, Crystal
Grids transcend space and time)).

So here you are at work, and guess what? That Crystal can no longer
assist you because you lost the connection.

I like to tell people to keep it on them! Whether it be a pocket, or
bra, somewhere close is best. You can usually get Crystals in jewelry
form (rings, bracelets, necklaces) so that is another way you can
receive their benefits. You can also have it in your purse, so long as
it's nearby you (don't leave it in your car).

⭕ Meditate

Another way you can work with your Crystals is meditate with them. Meditation is an amazing way to tap into their healing energy!

You can do this by closing your eyes, taking a few deep breaths and hold your Crystal.

Feel the Crystal's energy intermingle with yours. Sometimes you might feel a tingle, vibration, or a hovering sensation. Each Crystal will be different. As you meditate with them, you are allowing a deeper connection and friendship with them.

⭕ Lay On You

The best way to soak up Crystal energy is to place your Crystal on you. If you are trying to say relax a stomachache, you would place your Crystals (Tiger Eye, Yellow Calcite, Yellow Apatite) on your stomach (Solar Plexus).

As you lay with the Crystal on you, relax and feel it's loving energy heal the area.

When you are done working with your Crystal for healing your physical body, it's always a good idea to cleanse it and allow it a good recharge.

This way your Crystal will be ready to assist you again.

○ Crystal Elixirs

Crystal Elixirs are another way you can work with Crystals. An Elixir is basically water that is charged with Crystal energy. **Something to note, not all Crystals are good to put in water… and some can in fact be toxic!**

It's always wise to do your homework when it comes to Crystal Elixirs.
I will give you an example/recipe for a Crystal Elixir.

Say your goal is to achieve calmness, to relax, detox from stress.
I would work with an Amethyst Crystal for this.

First, cleanse your Crystal by smudging.
Then you would program your Crystal so that the Crystal had a direct focus as to what you'd like it to do to help you. If you don't program it, that's fine too…. I just have found better results when it has instructions as to what you want your outcome to be.

After you program, you would fill a glass bottle or bowl up with purified water.
Next, you wash off your Crystal in antibacterial soap just to make sure it's clean before putting it in water you will be ingesting.

Then carefully allow the Crystal to slide into the purified water. It's best to used tumbles stones for this purpose.

Next, hold the Crystal Elixir up to your 3rd eye and say your intention aloud something like this " Crystal Deva's please program this water with the intention of relaxation and calm." As you do this, envision how it will help you. See yourself drinking it, see how it brings a calming effect to you, and see yourself relaxed. The more clear you are in your visualization, the better the results.

It's a good idea to make sure your water is covered before placing it outside for the next step. Cover it with plastic wrap before leaving it outdoors, if you don't have a lid for it. You don't want anything to contaminate your Elixir!

Then, set your Crystal Elixir outside in either the Sun or Moon light. If you are trying to achieve energy, then place it in the Sun for a few hours. If you are trying to find peace and calm then the Moon light would be your best source. Place it outside and collect it in the morning.

<u>Keep in mind, it's a good idea to drink your Crystal Elixir with a straw so you don't accidentally ingest your Crystal!! We don't want to do that!</u>

If you are worried about swallowing your Crystal(s) and you don' have a straw, then after you are done charging it… you can remove the Crystal(s) before drinking.

There are many ideas and recipes for Crystal Elixirs I'll list a few ideas here.
All the recipes I list below are SAFE!

- Cold: *Carnelian*
- Connection to Sprit: *Clear Quartz*
- Remove Addiction : *Amethyst*
- Relaxation: *Amethyst*
- Boost Energy: *Carnelian or Citrine*
- Positivity: *Citrine*
- Boost Intuition: *Amethyst or Ametrine*
- Headache Relief: *Amethyst*

Programming Crystals

Programming/Setting Intentions for Crystals.

Crystals have many amazing capabilities to help us. As you learn more about Crystals you will see that just 1 Crystal has many ways of assisting. For example…Amethyst is great for relieving headaches, but it's also great for tapping into you intuition, helping you feel peace and calm, it's also good for someone who is ready to release addiction from their life. As you see, Amethyst has many ways of helping us.

By programming a Crystal or setting an intention for it, you're putting a laser focus on exactly what you're wanting the Crystal to help you with. So say you have a headache, you could program that Amethyst just to focus on removing any pain from the headache, allowing the Crystal Deva to know exactly what your wanting to get out of it.

Step by Step… Programming/Setting Intentions for Crystal(s):
1. CLEANSE: your Crystal (Sage/Palo Santo).
2. CHARGE: your Crystal (Sun/Moon Light).
3. MEDITATE: go into a meditative state, take a few deep breaths to clear your mind.
4. HOLD TO: your 3rd Eye and ask (either aloud or quietly to yourself) the Crystal Devas (the spirit within the Crystal) to please program this Crystal to help ______________(relieve my headache).
5. VISUALIZE: in as much detail as you can, visualize how this Crystal will help assist you in achieving your programed goal. The more details the better. See yourself placing the Crystal on your head (headache). See yourself enjoying the vibration of the Crystal. Feel yourself no longer in pain and in a relaxed state. And see yourself moving through the rest of your day happy and pain free.
6. GRATITUDE: thank the Crystal Deva for coming into your life and helping assist you. You can also thank anyone else you feel fit to do so. I usually thank the Crystal Devas, Spirit Guides, Spirit Animals, Universe, Sun, Moon, Stars, Elements. But, you don't have to get too wordy. Do what feels right to you, that's the beauty of it…it's not set in stone, you can do what works and feels right for you.

Now that you have programmed your Crystal there are a few things to know. One super important thing is that you should never share that Crystal with anyone else. That Crystal is now programmed to you for it's intention(s) you picked.

Also, if you are working with a Crystal to remove pain…I recommend cleansing and recharging it after use.

Remember, the pain has to go somewhere…it doesn't just disappear. The Crystal takes it on, thus if we don't properly cleanse and recharge it….it will not help us as it did at the beginning and you might feel like the Crystal "isn't working anymore"! If you ever have that feeling with any of your Crystals, it's time to cleanse them!

Say for example, you have enjoyed the benefits from that Amethyst Crystal to remove your headache, but now you'd like to have it's assistance with enhancing your intuition! Well then my friend, it's time to de-program your Crystal!

De-Programming Crystals

Once your ready to not work with that Crystal for the previous program you have selected, the Crystal needs to be de-programed.

When you cleanse the Crystal with Sage or Palo Santo, it will NOT remove any previously programmed intentions!! It only removes any of the energy it collected from you to help assist you. So when you are ready to work with the Crystal in a new way, you must take the time to de-program, or reset it!

Step by Step… de-programming or resetting your Crystal(s):
1. CLEANSE: your Crystal (Sage/Palo Santo).
2. CHARGE: your Crystal (Sun/Moon Light).
3. MEDITATE: go into a meditative state, take a few deep breaths to clear your mind.
4. HOLD ABOVE: your 3rd Eye, not on it. Ask (either aloud or quietly to yourself) the Crystal Devas (the spirit within the Crystal) to please remove and delete any previous programs, to please reset this Crystal to it's natural state of being.
5. VISUALIZE: white light coming into your Crown Chakra (top of your head) and entering down through you, into your Heart Chakra and out your hands. Sending an immense amount of light and love to that Crystal. Visualize the white loving light to remove any of the previous programs leaving it cleansed and reset to it's natural state.
6. GRATITUDE: thank the Crystal Deva for coming into your life and helping assist you. You can also thank anyone else you feel fit to do so. I usually thank the Crystal Devas, Spirit Guides, Spirit Animals, Universe, Sun, Moon, Stars, Elements. But, you don't have to get too wordy. Do what feels right to you, that's the beauty of it…it's not set in stone, you can do what works and feels right for you.

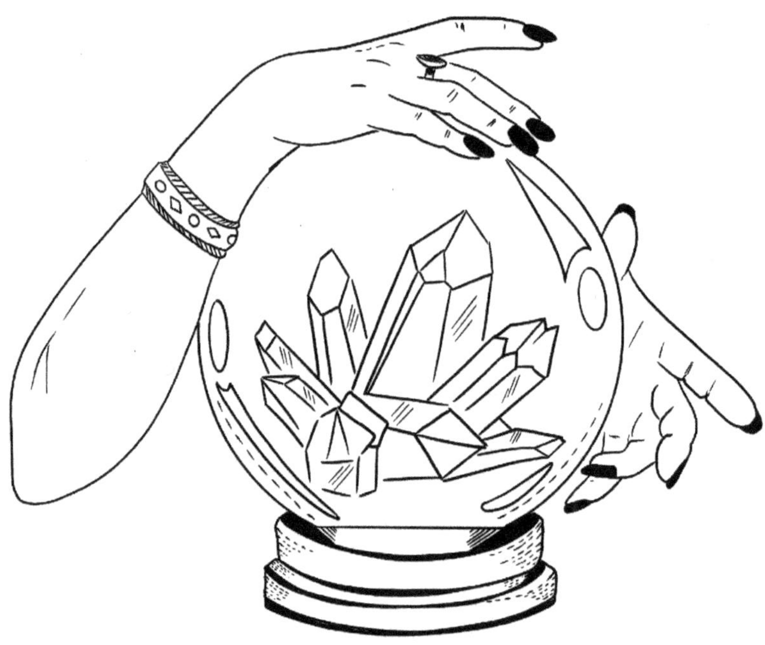

SECTION 3
MAGICKAL MINERALS
(FOR *WITCHES*)

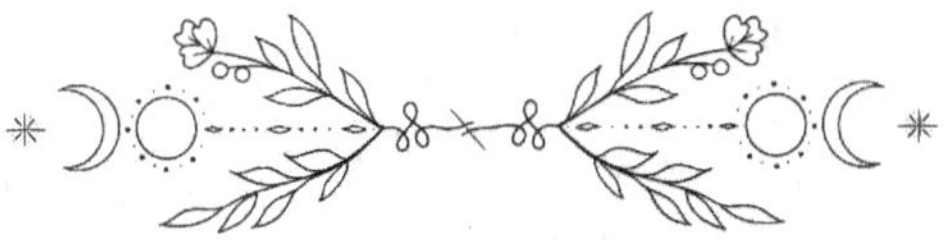

Crystals and Witches definitely go hand and hand. Witches have been crafting their magick with Crystals for centuries!

If you have ever held a Crystal in your hand, you can feel it's magick intermingling with yours!! There is no doubt that Crystals possess magick within them!

Just as the Ancient Egyptians worked with certain Crystals for protection, Witches also have a handful of Crystals they work with to amplify their magick spells.

Clear Quartz of course is one of the most common Crystals a Witch will work with. After all, that is what our Crystal balls are made of! It's the "go to" Crystal as it's the most versatile Crystals for Witches and people alike.

There are many ways we can work Crystals into our magick. Just like candle magick where each color of the candle offers a different vibration (like ingredients in a cake) to the spell. Crystals are the same!

Crystals are each so different in not only their visible looks, but how they can help assist our magick become more powerful!

Just as we did with working with Herbs for magickal use, the same are for Crystals.

You don't need to constantly think about it, allow the magick to bake within the belly of the Universe. It's the Universe's job to expand upon our magickal askings. All we have to do is stay in a high vibration, one of positive emotions.

Just as a reminder… it's like baking that cake we talked about earlier! When we put the cake into the oven, you don't open the door several times to check on it to make sure it's doing it's job? Nope! You simply trust and know that you put the work in, and a positive outcome will follow.

Consider this when doing your Magickal Spell work. Do your spells and then let them go, trusting in the Universal energies!

In this chapter I will cover some of my must have Crystals if you are a Witch. I will also share with you some of my favorite spells that incorporate Crystals!!

So… let's begin!

Must Have Minerals

As we learned earlier, there are over 4,000 different Minerals in the Mineral Kingdom and more and more discovered each day! With that being said, I won't be covering them all. I have compiled my Must have Minerals for Magickal purposes here. Now for me, picking and choosing which Minerals to list here is a challenge… for they are all my favorites and "must haves", it's almost like choosing which child you like best. You just can't! But I will do my best to share my Must have Minerals with you!

Clear Quartz

The Master Healer!! This Mineral Friend will be there for any and all things you could possibly think of. From healing your physical body, to boosting your energy, protection, or accelerating your desires, Clear Quartz has you covered!
Also beneficial in clearing your mind, connecting to Spirit, and amplifying your healing abilities.
Great for scrying… you know looking into your Crystal ball type magick!
Excellent at unlocking the abilities of the mind.

Amethyst

This purple beauty is a pretty common Mineral Friend. Most Witches have this loveliness all over either themselves, or their home.
Purple of course is associated with being a Witch, as this royal color is closely related to intuition, mysticism and the supernatural.

If you have ever been to my house, you have seen my Purple front door… an indicator that a "Witch Lives Here!" But also, to encourage having an open mind, and invites in opportunity and inspiration into our space.
Amethyst is great for protection, peace, and calmness, increases spiritual awareness, and enhances intuition. It's also great for relieving headaches!

Turquoise
Oh the blue amazing color of Turquoise. A prized possession for so many. This alluring Mineral has been worked with by Native American's for as far back as history dates. It is known metaphysically as the bridge between Heaven, Sky and Earth. Grounding us while still remaining open to Spirit.

Turquoise is amazing for connecting to your Spirit Guides, and understanding messages coming your way. Another marvelous Mineral for protection, and enhances your communication skills. Great for a beginner in spell and Divine workings. It gives you strength, vitality, and relieves pain. Also beneficial for lung or breathing issues.

Labradorite
The Mineral of Magick!
I don't know about you, but I'm a sucker for Crystal flash! You know when a Crystal has internal color that moves! Labradorite is known for it's lovely flash, or it's more scientific identification as feldspar. Basically there are layers within the Mineral that refract or reflect light which is known as labradorescence or what I call… Flash!

Unbelievably powerful in awakening your Magickal powers!
This is the Mineral of Magick as it brings forward your mystical and magickal abilities. Helps open your psychic powers and is also another great one for protection. It has the ability to protect your aura and the cool thing is, if you have any leaks in your aura… Labradorite will go straight to work and repair them for you!

This charming friends is also great for lowering blood pressure, regulating metabolism and banishes fear... allowing you to trust in yourself & Universe.

Shungite
This 2 billion year old Crystal comes all the way from Russia! Shungite is incredibly protective! Not only protecting your energetic body, but also your physical body as well. It has the ability to block EMF's (electromagnetic frequencies… given off from wifi, cell phones computers, tv's).
It can also boost your immune system, removes negativity from your environment, and rids your body of any colds/flu.

Beneficial in connecting you to the earth's energy, it also allows you to stay grounded which is important when you are working in the Spirit realm. It has a way of evolving you spiritually as you work with it as well.

Minerals and Magick

Here I will share a few of my personal spell workings.
Feel free to tweak them as you see fit.

The way I have written them has brought me success, but as every good Witch knows… it's best to go with your intuition and change anything that might call to you. This is especially true if you haven't come out of the "broom closet" yet! You can always modify the spells by working with a alternate Crystal in your collection.

My spells below are definitely not "set in stone."

That is the beauty of Witch craft, there is no "one size fits all".
You have the ability to craft together whatever style feels right to you.

So… hop on your broomstick and follow me!

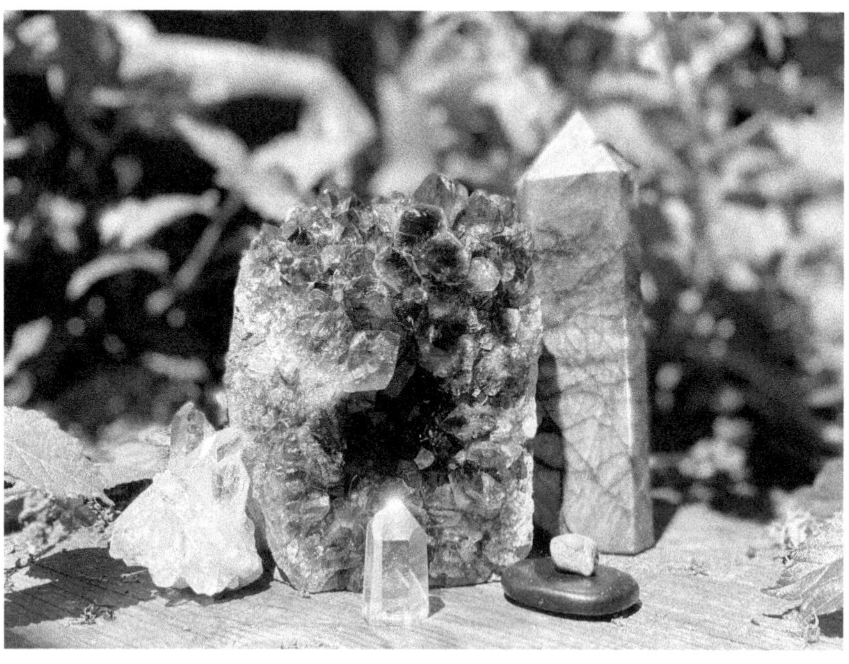

Magickal Money Spell

Items you will need:

- Citrine
- Small piece of paper
- 1 Dollar Bills (or any bill amount)

What to do:

Take a small piece of paper and write on it
"Money is flowing to me in all ways. I welcome this new feeling with ease and grace. As I find my happiness more abundant I will be, focus on the moments and choose to live carefree."

Fold the paper up.
Then take a small Citrine Crystal with the folded up paper with your intention and place them both in the center of the dollar bill.
Fold the dollar bill up and tie with a ribbon or yarn.
Charge your Magick Money Spell by holding the dollar bill in your hands, picture money flowing to you with ease. See your abundance.

Now take this dollar bill and place it in your wallet or next to your money, and watch as your money grows!

Magickal Protection Talisman

Items you will need:
- Clear Quartz point or any Crystal, (one you can put on a necklace) this is your talisman.
- Chain or cord
- Water
- Chalice, Bowl or Cup
- White or Silver Candle
- Moonlight or Sunlight

What to do:

After cleansing and charging your Clear Quartz Crystal. Go into a meditative state of relaxation & clear your mind.

Program your Crystal (see chapter 2/section 2) with the intention of protection.

See how this Clear Quartz Crystal will keep you safe and protected. The more you can visualize this clearly, the better the results.

Light your white candle to invite protection as you do your spell work.

Then pour a small amount of water in you Chalice.

Hold your hands over the Chalice and say: "Water from the West, please bring your blessed best, to charge this charm with protection and no harm."

Now it's time to recite your spell!

Holding your Clear Quartz Crystal in your hand say the following: "With this Crystal, I am safe and secure. Peace and Positivity I do endure.

As I travel, I'm protected in every single way. I give thanks to this Crystal who helps bring protection day by day. During the day or during the night, this Crystal will hold it's power of golden white protective light. And so it is so."

Now place your Crystal in the water and make sure it is covered completely.
Allow it to sit outside under the Moonlight and collect it in the morning. If you choose to charge by Sunlight, leave it out for at least 3 hours and then collect it.

Now your Clear Quartz Crystal will offer you Magickal protection at all times. Wear it as you travel or daily. This spell will last for 1 years time. After that, you will want to do this process again.

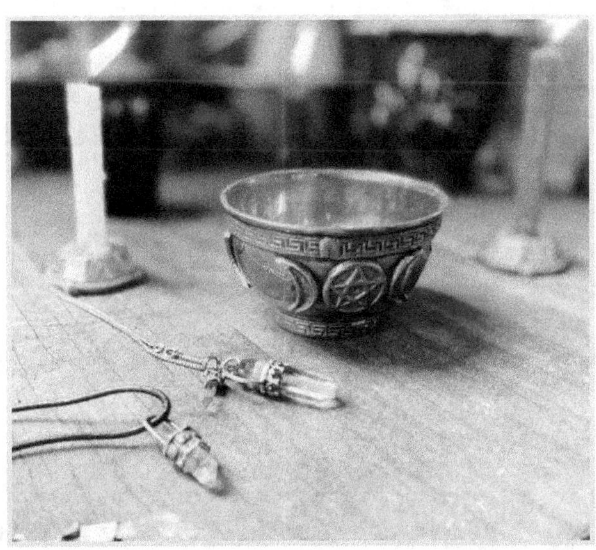

Magickal Cleansing Spell
Items you will need:
- Sage or Palo Santo
- Lighter/Matches
- Smudging Wand
- Abalone Shell
- Clear Quartz Crystal or Wand

What to do:
This cleansing spell will cleanse your space free of any low or negative vibrations!

Pick your method of smudge (Sage, Palo Santo, etc), with the lighter…light your method. Once it begins to smoke you will walk anti-clockwise around your space (home/office/room). Take your smudging wand and waft the smoke where you need it to go.

As you do this, you are picturing any low vibrations or negativity to leave this space with the smoke.

While you are circling your space say aloud:
"Negative energy please disappear, please get far far away from here. We have no space in our place, so we vanish you into outer space. The Universe will take care of you now, and turn you into positive energy for all around.
And with these words, I do say… Poof Be Gone and send you on your way,
And so it is so."

After you have cleansed all of the areas within your space, oh don't forget doorways, windows and stairs (lots of energy collects there).

Next you will place your smudging stick in the abalone shell to allow it to safely extinguish it's self.

Last up, take your Clear Quartz Crystal… or Crystal Wand.
Walk around your space again, making sure to draw a pentagram on each of the doorways. We do this to add an additional layer of protection to the space.

Magickal Vanishing Spell

Items you will need:

- Lepidolite
- Labradorite
- Amethyst

What to do:

This vanishing spell will allow you space and time to not be disturbed. I have used this spell successfully to not be seen by others when needing a few minutes to myself, or a group of people.

One thing to keep in mind, this spell has a time frame on it! Make sure that you are done with whatever it is you are doing, as for once the time has run out, you will no longer be invisible to the muggle (human) eye.

Take the Crystals I have mentioned above with you. If you don't have all three it's ok, pick the one that call to you.

I like to work with Lepidolite for calmness during this spell as if your energy is all over the place you can be detected.
Labradorite for protection, and Amethyst for increasing psychic awareness and tapping into your intuition.

Have the Crystals either on you or near you during the full hour.

Calm your mind by taking a few deep breaths. Relax!
Once you get into a deep relaxed state recite the following spell:

"This circle has vanished, there is nothing to see.
Everyone in this circle is unseen with me.
Just walk right past and move along,
the spell will be over when an hour is gone.
And so it is so."

After you have said these words, visualize how you, and or your group will not be disturbed during that hour. See what you will be doing with much success.

Then enjoy the hour distraction free!

Magickal Meditation Spell

Items you will need:
- Clear Quartz Crystal
- Sodalite Crystal
- Cleansed Space (see magickal cleansing spell)

What to do:

Find a place where you will be distraction free before you start your meditation.

This Magickal Meditation Spell will help you connect more deeply during your meditation. Whether it be a meet up with your Spirit Guides or loved ones from beyond. It could also be to enhance your meditation or connection with your higher self.
You get to choose!

Once you have found your location, cleanse your space of any low or negative vibrations. (see the Magickal Cleansing Spell)

Place your Crystals, one in each hand.
Relax your body and take a few deep breaths to release thoughts from your mind.

Then recite your spell:
"Meditation time is here, time to see things Crystal Clear.
My mind is settled & ready to receive,
I'm open to new downloads to help me perceive.
Time to reflect during my introspect… it's my quiet time to reconnect.
Today I say Namaste, and get my meditation on it's way.
And so it is so."

Then continue to connect to whom ever you'd like during your meditation.
Enjoy!

SECTION 4
HEALING WITH CRYSTALS

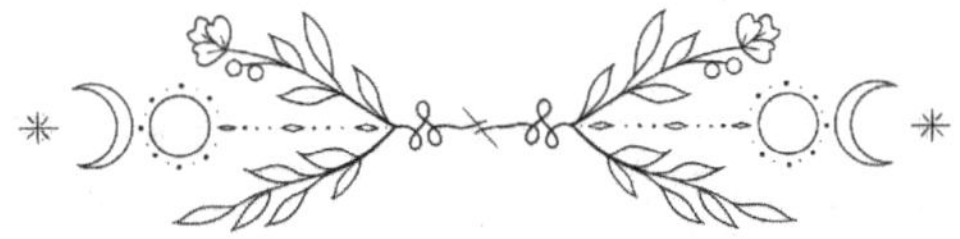

In this chapter you will get to discover the fascinating healing powers of Crystals!

As I had mentioned earlier in this book, Crystals have helped heal myself and my family time and time again!

This list that I will be providing in this chapter is just what I have found most people might need assistance with in the healing department.

Whether it be healing your physical body, mental body, emotional body, or spiritual body…. you will get to discover how to heal them all.

It's always best to find a reputable Crystal dealer when purchasing your new Mineral friends. If you are ever in need, you can always reach out to me as I do sell my Crystals in my "Gypsy Crystal Shop". This is my little Crystal shop that travels with me when I see my Clients!

I handpick my Crystals, so I always look for the best of the best!

One online shop that is a personal friend and favorite of mine is "The Crystal Angel". She is on Etsy and also vends at the Crystal Conventions.
You can order online from her here:
(https://www.etsy.com/shop/TheCrystalAngel888)

Friendly reminder that anytime you receive or purchase a Crystal, make sure you clean and charge them before your 1st use. Make sure you always are mindful about cleansing after working with a Crystal so that Crystal friends will be ready to assist you in the future.

One thing to note is that Clear Quartz Crystals are the master healers and can help heal any and all ailments. I won't be listing them in each ailment topic, but just know if that is the only Crystal you have… it will do just fine!

Ways to work with Crystals for Healing

Carry them on you
As you carry them on you they will entrain with your body and allow you to soak up their pure positive high vibration. Which in turn will help heal your body!

Place them on you
Allowing the Crystal to be on the space you are trying to heal will help heal it! If you are using a Crystal with a point, it matters how you hold or place the Crystal on you. You must know which way the point should face! Remember... "Where the point goes, energy flows."

Therefore, if say you had knee pain... I would recommend a Smokey Quartz point. You would place it on your knee with the point of the Crystal pointing down your leg and towards your foot.

The reason why we do this is that we don't want any of the low painful vibrations to travel up our energetic body (chakras). By allowing it to escape in the quickest, but also away from our chakras as much as possible is the most beneficial.

Keep in mind, you can always heal any part of your body with a Clear Quartz Crystal. I love working with my Clear Quartz Crystal point to remove any neck pain, or shoulder pain from myself. Again looking for the fastest escape route, I usually place it on my neck with the point facing up towards the top of my head.

Crystal Elixirs
I touched on this earlier in the book. I'm not going to focus too much on this subject. The reason why is that not all Crystals can go into a Crystal Elixir and be safe to ingest.

The basics on how to make a Crystal Elixir is found in (chapter 2/section 2).

Please do your own research to make sure the Crystal you are going to work with for your Crystal Elixir is safe!!

Know that <u>ALL</u> in the <u>Quartz</u> family <u>ARE SAFE</u> Crystals for Elixirs:
- Clear Quartz
- Rose Quartz
- Smokey Quartz
- Amethyst
- Citrine
- Ametrine

How to work with this list:

In the Crystal list to follow, you can look up the ailment you'd like to focus your healing attention on. I will list the Crystals that I have found to work great for that ailment. You will notice there is more than one Crystal listed, try working with one at a time to see which one is the best fit for you.

The following information will be included:
- Healing Use
- Emotional Use
- Spiritual Use
- Chakra
- Moh's Hardness
- Zodiac
- Water Safety

Just note, the Chakra information will help you know which Chakra that particular Crystal works best with.

The Moh's Hardness is the hardness of each Crystal.

In Zodiac, I will list the zodiac signs that is closely linked to the Crystal. What that means is the zodiac sign listed… that Crystal will help balance out that zodiac's positive and negative qualities within those signs. If your zodiac Sun or Moon sign isn't listed, it doesn't mean you can't work with that Crystal. All it means is that particular Crystal helps bring more balance to that zodiac sign(s).

Water Safety is important, especially if you decide to start dabbling in making your own Crystal Elixirs. I will mention if the Crystal is safe for water in the following list too.

Sometimes it's nice to put the Crystal with you in your bath water! For example.. Rose Quartz is great to bring peace and calm, but bonus it helps rid you of wrinkles! That one is safe for water.

So, when I list the water safety and it says "yes", that means it's safe to put that Crystal in water. Whether it be to cleanse it, to bathe with it… or place in a Crystal Elixir. <u>Again, please work with Crystals for Elixirs with caution! Also double check that Crystal is safe before working with it in an Elixir!</u>

A Word of Caution:
Crystals will NOT interact in a negative way if you are taking prescription drugs or Herbs. In fact, I would encourage you to work with Crystals & Herbs together!

However, Crystal healing and other types of energy work are not to be considered as a substitute for conventional medicine.
If you have a serous health issue, you should consult your doctor and make energy healing part of a complete health care program.

My Crystal List is in alphabetical order based on the ailment. You might notice a lot of the same Crystals are used for many ailments!

At the back of the book in the index, I will list the Crystals by name and it's page number so you can reference all the ailments that particular Crystal will assist with.

Ok. let's get to the list!

Crystal List

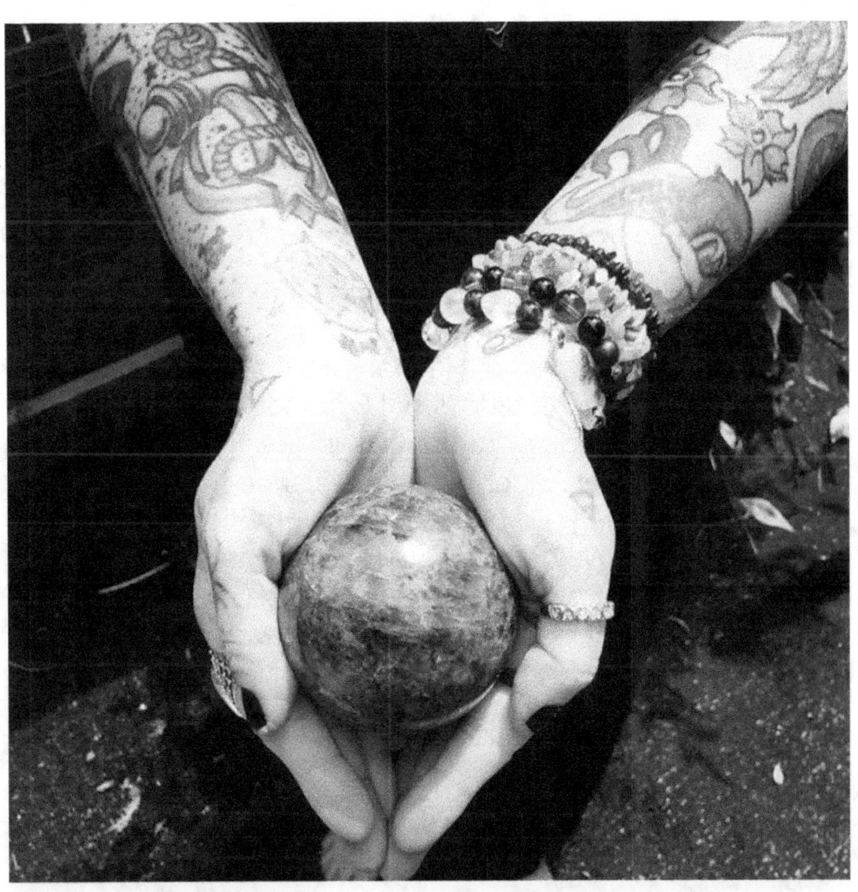

To Assist You In The Healing Process!

-A-

ADHD
Other Crystals To Try: Amethyst, Lepidolite, Hematite, Amazonite, Rose Quartz

Amethyst
- ✦ **Healing Use:** ADHD, Focus, Calm, Intuition, Addiction, Acne, Alcoholism, Bruises, Burns, Cancer, Digestion, Dreams, Ears, Eczema, Headaches, Insomnia, Itching, Lungs, Memory, Metabolism, Migraines, Nightmares, Pain, Psoriasis, Skin, Tumors, Wrinkles.
- ✦ **Emotional Use:** Anger, Anxiety, Balance, Coping, Decision Making, Dispel Negativity, Emotional Pain, Fear, Grief, Loss, Love, Motivation, Reduce Stress, Serenity
- ✦ **Spiritual Use:** Astral Travel, Awareness, Dream Recall, Harmony, Higher Self, Intuition, Love, Mediation, Mediumship, Protection, Psychic Abilities, Telekinesis, Visitation, Wisdom
- ✦ **Chakra:** Third Eye
- ✦ **Moh's Hardness:** 7
- ✦ **Zodiac:** Aquarius/Capricorn/Pisces/Virgo
- ✦ **Safe for Water:** Yes

<u>ALLERGIES</u>
Other Crystals To Try: Moss Agate, Carnelian, Red Jasper

Moss Agate
✦ **Healing Use:** Allergies, Virus, Bacterial Infection, Backache, Crohn's, Digestion, Birthing
✦ **Emotional Use:** Calming, Calming for Animals, Compassion, Mood Swings, Relationships, Soothing, Abundance, Depression
✦ **Spiritual Use:** Communication w/Animals & Plants, Healing, Earth Healing
✦ **Chakra:** Heart
✦ **Moh's Hardness:** 6-7
✦ **Zodiac:** Virgo
✦ **Safe for Water:** Yes

ALZHEMIER'S

Other Crystals To Try: Rhodonite, Rutilated Quartz, Rose Quartz, Lepidolite

Rhodonite
- ✦ **Healing Use:** Alzheimer's, Memory, Arthritis, Autoimmune Disorder, Burns, Cancer, Ears, Heart, Insect Bites, Joints, MS
- ✦ **Emotional Use:** Emotional Balance, Forgiveness, Harmony, Kindness, Self Love
- ✦ **Spiritual Use:** Insight, Unconditional Love
- ✦ **Chakra:** Heart
- ✦ **Moh's Hardness:** 5.5-6.5
- ✦ **Zodiac:** Taurus
- ✦ **Safe for Water:** Yes

Rutilated Quartz
- ✦ **Healing Use:** Memory, Clear Mind, Body Balance, Bronchitis, Cellular Disorders, Impotence, Food Poisoning, Lactating, Smoking Addiction, Veins
- ✦ **Emotional Use:** Building Relationships, Intuition
- ✦ **Spiritual Use:** Astral Travel, Astral Projection, Cleanses Aura, Clairsentience, Meditation
- ✦ **Chakra:** Crown/Third Eye
- ✦ **Moh's Hardness:** 6-6.5
- ✦ **Zodiac:** Gemini/Taurus
- ✦ **Safe for Water:** Yes

ANEMIA

Other Crystals To Try: Bloodstone, Hematite, Tiger's Eye, Garnet, Copper

Bloodstone
✦ **Healing Use:** Anemia, Boost Immune System, Blood Detoxifying, Bone Marrow, Bronchitis, Heart, High Blood Pressure, Tumor, Stops Bleeding, Colon, Cramps
✦ **Emotional Use:** Anger, Courage, Compassion, Grounding, Unselfishness
✦ **Spiritual Use:** Awareness, Humility, Prosperity, Serving Humanity
✦ **Chakra:** Heart/Root
✦ **Moh's Hardness:** 7
✦ **Zodiac:** Aries/Libra/Pisces
✦ **Safe for Water:** No

ANXIETY

Other Crystals To Try: Lepidolite, Amethyst, Blue Laced Agate, Chrysoprase, Sunstone

Lepidolite

- ✦ **Healing Use:** ADHD, ADD, Stress, Anxiety, Panic Attacks, Insomnia, Alzheimer's ,Epilepsy, Allergies, Anorexia, Menopause, Night Terror, Nightmares, Schizophrenia, Stomach
- ✦ **Emotional Use:** Anxiety, Stress, Depression, PTSD, Balances Emotions, Bipolar, Mood Swings, Rage, Relaxing, Tension
- ✦ **Spiritual Use:** Akashic Records, Balances Yin, Cosmic Awareness, Electromagnetic Pollution
- ✦ **Chakra:** Heart/Third Eye/Crown
- ✦ **Moh's Hardness:** 2.5-3
- ✦ **Zodiac:** Libra
- ✦ **Safe for Water:** No

<u>ARTHRITIS</u>

Other Crystals To Try: Azurite, Fluorite, Malachite, Rhodonite, Copper

Azurite

- ✦ **Healing Use:** Arthritis, Asthma, Blood Disorders, Brain Disorder, Congestion, Hip Pain, Itching, Joint Pain, Legs, Liver, Sinus, Spleen, Thyroid, Tinnitus
- ✦ **Emotional Use:** Comforting, Kindness, Patience, Decision Making, Self Confidence, Self Worth, Worry
- ✦ **Spiritual Use:** Balances Aura, Clairvoyance, Communication with Higher Self, Cosmic Awareness
- ✦ **Chakra:** Throat/Third Eye
- ✦ **Moh's Hardness:** 3.5-4
- ✦ **Zodiac:** Aquarius/Sagittarius
- ✦ **Safe for Water:** No

ASTHMA
Other Crystals To Try: Amber, Tiger's Eye, Rose Quartz, Jade

Amber
✦ **Healing Use:** Asthma, Arthritis, Cold, Flu, Bone Disorders, Breathing Issues, Dental Pain, Gallbladder, Headache, Boosts Immune System, Infection, Intestinal Disorders, Kidney Issues, Nervous System, Pancreas, Pneumonia, Pregnancy, Skin Issues, Throat, UTI, Constipation, Ovarian Disorders
✦ **Emotional Use:** Centering, Releases Negativity, Eases Depression, Grounding, Patience, Stress, Anxiety
✦ **Spiritual Use:** Ancient Knowledge, Balances Aura, Clairsentience, Earth Healing, Past Life Recall
✦ **Chakra:** Solar Plexus
✦ **Moh's Hardness:** 2-2.5
✦ **Zodiac:** Aquarius/Leo
✦ **Safe for Water:** No

Tiger's Eye
✦ **Healing Use:** Asthma, Bronchitis, Insomnia, Fatigue, Night Vision, Broken Bones, Throat, Balances Brain Hemispheres
✦ **Emotional Use:** Boost Personal Power, Depression, Mental Illness, Self Worth, Lifts Mood
✦ **Spiritual Use:** Protection During Travel, Growth, Peace, Beauty, Connects with Spiritual Power, Joy
✦ **Chakra:** Solar Plexus
✦ **Moh's Hardness:** 7
✦ **Zodiac:** Capricorn/Leo
✦ **Safe for Water:** No

AUTISM

Other Crystals To Try: Blue Apatite, Tigers Eye, Red Jasper, Jade, Charoite

Blue Apatite
- ✦ **Healing Use:** Autism, Hyperthyroidism, Appetite suppressant, Brings Body into Balance, Renews Body
- ✦ **Emotional Use:** Inspiration, Helping Others, Clarity of Mind, Enhances Communication, Self Expression, Emotional openness, Balances Emotions
- ✦ **Spiritual Use:** Cleanse Aura, Balances Chakras, Balances Yin/Yang Energies, Helps you Uncover the Truth, Develop Psychic Gifts, Meditation, Clairvoyance, Clairaudience
- ✦ **Chakra:** Throat
- ✦ **Moh's Hardness:** 5
- ✦ **Zodiac:** Gemini/Libra
- ✦ **Safe for Water:** No

-B-

BACTERIA INFECTION
Other Crystals To Try: Green Calcite

Green Calcite
- ✦ **Healing Use:** Bacteria Infection, Virus, Arthritis, Bladder Issues, Regulates Body Temp, Burns, Fever, Heartburn, Boost Immune System, Joint Pain, Tumors, Skin Infections
- ✦ **Emotional Use:** Anxiety, Balances Emotions, Panic Attacks, Rage, Worry, Releases Stress
- ✦ **Spiritual Use:** Abundance, Balance, Communication
- ✦ **Chakra:** Heart
- ✦ **Moh's Hardness:** 2.5-3
- ✦ **Zodiac:** Cancer/Virgo
- ✦ **Safe for Water:** No

BIPOLAR DISORDER
Other Crystals To Try: Snowflake Obsidian, Lepidolite, Charorite, Kunzite

Snowflake Obsidian
✦ **Healing Use:** Balances Body, Abdominal Problems, Digestion, Ear Infection, Hearing Issues, Skin Infections
✦ **Emotional Use:** Calming, Soothing, Loneliness, Dispels Anger, Releases Wrong Thinking
✦ **Spiritual Use:** Balances Mind, Body and Soul, Astral Travel, Dispels Negativity, Protection, Transformation
✦ **Chakra:** Root
✦ **Moh's Hardness:** 5-5.5
✦ **Zodiac:** Virgo/Capricorn
✦ **Safe for Water:** No

Kunzite
✦ **Healing Use:** Brian Disorder, Addiction, Anemia, Dying Process/Transition, Epilepsy, Boosts Immune System, Inflammation, Swollen Joints, Lungs, Swelling, Throat
✦ **Emotional Use:** Bipolar Disorder, Calming, Eases Depression, Emotional Abuse, Balances Emotions, Gentleness, Kindness, Love, Self Love, Self Confidence, Self Worth, Soothing, Unconditional Love
✦ **Spiritual Use:** Meditation, Soul Retrieval, Divine Love, Connection to Guidance, Intuition, Creativity
✦ **Chakra:** Heart
✦ **Moh's Hardness:** 6.5-7
✦ **Zodiac:** Aries/Leo/Libra/Scorpio/Taurus
✦ **Safe for Water:** No

BLOOD PRESSURE (see hypertension)

BOOST MEMORY (see Alzheimer's)

BRUISING

Other Crystals To Try: Hematite, Angelite, Fluorite

Hematite
- ✦ **Healing Use:** Bruising, Anemia, Back issues, Addiction, Aids in Concentration, Circulatory Issues, Broken Bones, Cleanse Blood, Blood Clotting, Detoxifying, Focus, Nose Bleeds, Sclerosis, Leg Cramps, Menstrual Cramps, MS, Helps You Absorb Nutrients, Pain Relief, Strength, Heals Tissues
- ✦ **Emotional Use:** Diffuses Anger, Courage, Releases Negativity, Balances Emotions, Self Confidence, Self Worth
- ✦ **Spiritual Use:** Releases Negative Energy, Awareness, Balance, Stability, Growth, Harmony
- ✦ **Chakra:** Root
- ✦ **Moh's Hardness:** 5-6
- ✦ **Zodiac:** Aquarius/Aries
- ✦ **Safe for Water:** No

<u>BURSITIS</u>
Other Crystals To Try: Copper, Clear Quartz

Copper
✦ **Healing Use:** Joint Pain, Arthritis, Anemia, Bacteria/Viral Infections, Balances Metabolism, Blood Disorder, Balances Body, Bone Disorders, Circulatory Issues, Detoxifying, Exhaustion, Infection, Infertility
✦ **Emotional Use:** Calming, Self Confidence, Self Worth, Healthy Boundaries
✦ **Spiritual Use:** Abundance, Balance, Clarity, Prosperity, Protection
✦ **Chakra:** Root/Sacral
✦ **Moh's Hardness:** 2.5-3
✦ **Zodiac:** Sagittarius/ Taurus
✦ **Safe for Water:** No

-C-

CANCER

Other Crystals To Try: Citrine, Amethyst, Smokey Quartz, Emerald, Carnelian

Citrine

- ✦ **Healing Use:** Cancer, Diabetes, Circulatory Issues, Digestive Issues, Food Poisoning, Gallbladder, Headache, Migraine, Kidney Issues, Pancreas, Spleen, Balances Thyroid
- ✦ **Emotional Use:** Hope, Happiness, Courage, Creativity, Releases Negativity, Honesty, Hope, Inspiration, Joy, Self Confidence, Self Worth, Shyness, Suicidal Thoughts
- ✦ **Spiritual Use:** Abundance, Manifestation, Enhances Psychic Abilities, Increases Energy Flow, Phobias, White Light, Releases Negativity
- ✦ **Chakra:** Solar Plexus/Sacral
- ✦ **Moh's Hardness:** 7
- ✦ **Zodiac:** Aries/Gemini/Leo/Libra
- ✦ **Safe for Water:** Yes

<u>CHOLESTROL (HIGH)</u>
Other Crystals To Try: Green Aventurine, Fluorite

Green Aventurine
✦ **Healing Use:** Heart Issues, Lowers Cholesterol, Eye Disorders, Healing, Vision, Health
✦ **Emotional Use:** Calming, Anxiety, Emotional Healing, Increases Positivity, Releases Rage, Stress, Soothing, Good Luck
✦ **Spiritual Use:** Abundance, Healing, Connection to Divine & Nature
✦ **Chakra:** Heart
✦ **Moh's Hardness:** 7
✦ **Zodiac:** Aries
✦ **Safe for Water:** Yes

CONSTIPATION

Other Crystals To Try: Ruby, Citrine, Amber, Red Jasper

Ruby

✦ **Healing Use:** Constipation, Diarrhea, Ulcers, UTI, Wounds, Anemia, Blood Circulation, Blood Clotting, Blood Pressure, Brain Disorder, Fever, Heart, Infertility, Intestinal Disorder, Kidney Issues, Legs, Menopause, Menstrual Cramps, Pineal Gland, PMS, Pregnancy, Reproductive Organs, Skin Issues, Stomach Issues

✦ **Emotional Use:** Happiness, Courage, Inspiration, Passion, Releases Negativity, Emotional Balance, Trust, Self Confidence, Self Worth

✦ **Spiritual Use:** Abundance, Long Distance Healing, Removes Negativity, Strengthens Aura

✦ **Chakra:** Heart/Root

✦ **Moh's Hardness:** 9

✦ **Zodiac:** Aries/Cancer/Leo/Sagittarius/Scorpio

✦ **Safe for Water:** No

COMMON COLD

Other Crystals To Try: Carnelian, Ametrine, Moss Agate, Emerald

Carnelian
- **Healing Use:** Cold, Flu, Allergies, Appetite Control, Asthma, Back Issues, Blood Disorders, Detoxes Body, Edema, Gallbladder, Infection, Infertility, Intestinal Disorder, Kidney Issues, Liver Issues, Low Blood Pressure, Memory Health, Ovarian Disorder, Pain Relief, Scoliosis, UTI, Weakness
- **Emotional Use:** Self Confidence, Self Worth, Acceptance, Diffuses Anger, Courage, Comfort, Happiness, Understanding Death
- **Spiritual Use:** Balance, Past Life Recall, Reincarnation, Appreciation, Serenity, Spiritual Protection
- **Chakra:** Sacral
- **Moh's Hardness:** 7
- **Zodiac:** Cancer/Taurus
- **Safe for Water:** Yes

Ametrine
- **Healing Use:** Cold, Balances Metabolism, Immune System Strengthener, Jaundice, Mental Clarity, Ulcers, Exhaustion, Fatigue, Circulatory Issues, Balancing Issues, Alzheimer's, AIDS/HIV, Helps You Concentrate
- **Emotional Use:** Self Worth, Self Confidence, Anger, Anxiety, Grief Coping, Creativity, Decision Making, Fear, Motivation, Phobias
- **Spiritual Use:** Mental Clarity, Spiritual Protection, Transformation, Astral Travel/Projection, Meditation, Connecting with Higher Self, Psychic Awareness
- **Chakra:** Third Eye/Solar Plexus/Crown
- **Moh's Hardness:** 7
- **Zodiac:** Libra
- **Safe for Water:** Yes

COUGH

Other Crystals To Try: Blue Laced Agate, Amber, Aquamarine, Rose Quartz

Blue Laced Agate
- ✦ **Healing Use:** Cold, Flu, Cough, Abdominal Issues, Wounds, Pain, Arthritis, Asthma, Brain Disorder, Bruising, Dental Pain, Eye Disorder, Infections, Laryngitis, Poison, Psoriasis, Shingles, Sinus, Skin Infections, Stuttering, Tonsillitis, Ulcers, UTI
- ✦ **Emotional Use:** Peace, Sedative, Releases Anger, Anxiety, Conflict, Crying, Frustration, Honesty, Hope, Sedative
- ✦ **Spiritual Use:** Meditation, Communication with Spirit Guides, Angel Communication, Appreciation, Cleansing
- ✦ **Chakra:** Throat
- ✦ **Moh's Hardness:** 6-7
- ✦ **Zodiac:** Pisces
- ✦ **Safe for Water:** Yes

CROHN'S DISEASE

Other Crystals To Try: Chrysocolla, Hawk's Eye (Blue Tigers Eye), Yellow Jasper, Peridot, Green Aventurine, Blue Chalcedony

Chrysocolla
- ✦ **Healing Use:** Intestinal Issues, IBD, Ulcers, Arthritis, Breathing Issues, Bronchitis, Increases Metabolism, Leg Cramps, Lungs, Menstrual Cramps, Muscle Pain, Nervous System, Pancreas, PMS, Prostate Health
- ✦ **Emotional Use:** Hope, Joy, Gratitude, Balances Emotions, Releases Anger, Acceptance, Guilt, Trust, Kindness, Patience, Peace, Reduces Stress, Relationships
- ✦ **Spiritual Use:** Serenity, Meditation
- ✦ **Chakra:** Heart/Throat
- ✦ **Moh's Hardness:** 2-3.5
- ✦ **Zodiac:** Gemini/Taurus/Virgo
- ✦ **Safe for Water:** No

Hawk's Eye (Blue Tigers Eye)
- ✦ **Healing Use:** Balances Metabolism, Fatigue, Focus, Animal Healing, Clarity, Public Speaking, Eye Disorders, Libido
- ✦ **Emotional Use:** Emotional Balance, Honestly, Letting Go, Reduces Stress, Calming, Communication, Dignity, Eases Depression
- ✦ **Spiritual Use:** Enhances Intuition, Insight, Universal Love & Truth, Opens Aura, Clarity
- ✦ **Chakra:** Third Eye/Throat
- ✦ **Moh's Hardness:** 7
- ✦ **Zodiac:** Capricorn/Leo
- ✦ **Safe for Water:** No

-D-

<u>DEMENTIA (see Alzheimer's)</u>

<u>DEPRESSION (see anxiety)</u>

<u>DIABETES</u>
Other Crystals To Try: Pink Opal, Citrine, Emerald, Jade

Pink Opal
- ✦ **Healing Use:** Diabetes, Circulatory Issues, Low Blood Pressure, Skin Infections, Tension
- ✦ **Emotional Use:** Love, Grounding, Stress, Self Confidence, Self Worth, Tranquillity, Centering, Compassion
- ✦ **Spiritual Use:** Spiritual Awakening, Releasing Toxic Pattern, Divine Love, Connection with Spirit
- ✦ **Chakra:** Heart
- ✦ **Moh's Hardness:** 5.5-6
- ✦ **Zodiac:** Cancer/Libra/Pisces/Scorpio
- ✦ **Safe for Water:** No

-E-

ECZEMA

Other Crystals To Try: Fluorite, Amethyst, Green Aventurine

Fluorite

- ✦ **Healing Use:** Eczema, Pain Relief, Toothache, Gallbladder, ADD, ADHD, Arthritis, Bone Issues, Eating Disorders, Focus, Kidney Issues, Lungs, Improves Memory, Muscle Toning, Pneumonia, Sinus, Spleen, Virus, Ulcers
- ✦ **Emotional Use:** Honestly, Emotional Balance, Release Negativity, Denial
- ✦ **Spiritual Use:** Manifestation, Increases Intuition, Grounding, Stabilizes Aura, Higher Self, Awakening
- ✦ **Chakra:** Third Eye/Crown/Throat
- ✦ **Moh's Hardness:** 4
- ✦ **Zodiac:** Capricorn/Pisces
- ✦ **Safe for Water:** No

ERECTILE DISFUNCTION

Other Crystals To Try: Sunstone, Variscite, Carnelian, Rose Quartz

Sunstone

✦ **Healing Use:** Sexual issues, Aches, Pain, Stomach Tension, Ulcers, Digestion, Feet, Kidneys, Liver
✦ **Emotional Use:** Joy, Happiness, Harmony, Empowerment, Encouragement, Abundance, Leadership
✦ **Spiritual Use:** Aura Cleanser, Right use of Will, Good Luck
✦ **Chakra:** Sacral
✦ **Moh's Hardness:** 6-6.5
✦ **Zodiac:** Leo/Libra
✦ **Safe for Water:** No

EPILEPSY

Other Crystals To Try: Red Jasper, Amethyst, Black Tourmaline, Lapis Lazuli

Red Jasper
- ✦ **Healing Use:** Epilepsy, Vertigo, Vitality, Weakness, Physical Protection, Menstrual Cramps, Low Blood Pressure, Liver, Libido, Body Temp Regulator, Cancer, Circulatory Issues, Dizziness
- ✦ **Emotional Use:** Grounding
- ✦ **Spiritual Use:** Kundalini Energy, Dream Recall, Dream Interpretation
- ✦ **Chakra:** Root
- ✦ **Moh's Hardness:** 7
- ✦ **Zodiac:** Aries/Taurus
- ✦ **Safe for Water:** Yes

-F-

FEVER

Other Crystals To Try: Blue Chalcedony, Hematite, Carnelian

Blue Chalcedony
- ✦ **Healing Use:** Body Temperature, Throat Infections, IBS, Increases Lactation, Alzheimer's, Dementia, Gallstones, Tourette's
- ✦ **Emotional Use:** Calming, Communication, Creativity, Eases Depression
- ✦ **Spiritual Use:** Angel Communication, Connection To Spirit, Cleansing
- ✦ **Chakra:** Throat/Third Eye
- ✦ **Moh's Hardness:** 7
- ✦ **Zodiac:** Cancer/Sagittarius
- ✦ **Safe for Water:** Yes

FIBROMYALGIA

Other Crystals To Try: Malachite, Amethyst, Emerald, Hematite, Black Tourmaline, Clear Quartz

Malachite

✦ **Healing Use:** Fibromyalgia, Joints, Aches, Pain, Arthritis, Back Pain, Sciatica, Asthma, Bacterial/Viral Infections, Birthing, Cancer, Chemotherapy, Childbirth, Colic, Congestion, Dizziness, Headaches, Boost Immune System, Infection, Infertility, Inflammation, Itching, Liver, Lungs, Migraine, Osteoporosis, Rheumatism, Scoliosis, Tumor, Vertigo

✦ **Emotional Use:** Comfort, Balances Emotions, Hope, Shyness, Timid, Amplifies Positive/Negative, Draws out Negativity

✦ **Spiritual Use:** Absorbs Energy, Abundance, Manifestation, Psychic Vision (when placed on 3rd eye)

✦ **Chakra:** Heart

✦ **Moh's Hardness:** 3.5-4

✦ **Zodiac:** Capricorn/Scorpio

✦ **Safe for Water:** No

<u>FLU</u>

Other Crystals To Try: Labradorite, Moss Agate

Labradorite

✦ **Healing Use:** Regulates Metabolism, Flu, Eye Disorder, Brain Disorder, Gout, Rheumatism, Menstrual Cramps, Lowers Blood Pressure, Warts

✦ **Emotional Use:** Banishes Fear, Relieves Stress, Strengthens Faith In Self, Trust in Universe

✦ **Spiritual Use:** Aligns Physical & Etheric Bodies, Access to Spiritual Purpose, Stimulates Intuition, Protects Aura

✦ **Chakra:** Third Eye

✦ **Moh's Hardness:** 6-6.5

✦ **Zodiac:** Sagittarius/Scorpio/Leo

✦ **Safe for Water:** No

FREQUENT URINATION

Other Crystals To Try: Black Obsidian, Dragon's Eye (Red Tiger's Eye)

Black Obsidian
- ✦ **Healing Use:** Urinary Tract, Arthritis, Blockages, Joint Pain, Circulatory Issues, Detoxifying, Knee, Pain Relief, Physical Protection
- ✦ **Emotional Use:** Removes Emotional Blockages, Reduces Stress, Reduces Tension
- ✦ **Spiritual Use:** Grounding, Positive Vibrations, Energy, Psychic Protection
- ✦ **Chakra:** Root
- ✦ **Moh's Hardness:** 5-5.5
- ✦ **Zodiac:** Aries/Capricorn/Sagittarius/Scorpio
- ✦ **Safe for Water:** Yes

Dragon's Eye (Red Tiger's Eye)
- ✦ **Healing Use:** Urinary Tract, Increases Sexual Drive, Sexual Disfunction, Blood Disorders, Anemia, Eye Infections, Night Vision, Strength, Vitality
- ✦ **Emotional Use:** Calming, Enthusiasm, Motivation, Self Confidence, Balance, Unconditional Love
- ✦ **Spiritual Use:** Clarity
- ✦ **Chakra:** Root
- ✦ **Moh's Hardness:** 7
- ✦ **Zodiac:** Aries/Leo/Scoprio/Taurus
- ✦ **Safe for Water:** No

-G-

GALLBLADDER

Other Crystals To Try: Danburite, Carnelian, Amber, Citrine

Danburite
- ✦ **Healing Use:** Gallbladder, Infertility, Liver Disorders, Allergies, Body Detoxifier, Body Weight Management, Muscular, Tissues, Tumors
- ✦ **Emotional Use:** Comforting, Love, Patience, Peace, Reduces Stress, Sense of Belonging, Coping with Change
- ✦ **Spiritual Use:** Reiki, Truth, Raising Vibration, Psychic Work, Angel Communication, Aura Opening, Revitalizes Aura, Enhances Intuition, Protection
- ✦ **Chakra:** Heart/Crown
- ✦ **Moh's Hardness:** 7-7.5
- ✦ **Zodiac:** Leo
- ✦ **Safe for Water:** Yes

GOUT

Other Crystals To Try: Chrysoprase, Prehnite, Chaistolite, Labradorite

Chrysoprase
✦ **Healing Use:** Gout, Cramps, Menstrual Cramps, Heart, Low Blood Pressure, Digestion, Detoxifying, Prostate Health, Stone of Youth
✦ **Emotional Use:** Anxiety, Confidence, Self Worth, Positive Energy, Honesty, Hope, Happiness, Emotional Balance, Choice Making, Compromise
✦ **Spiritual Use:** Selflessness, Humility, Insight, Meditation, Connect with Inner Child
✦ **Chakra:** Heart
✦ **Moh's Hardness:** 7
✦ **Zodiac:** Libra/Taurus
✦ **Safe for Water:** Yes

Prehnite
✦ **Healing Use:** Gout, Bladder Issues, Body Detoxifier, Balances Energy, Addiction, Kidney Issues, Lymphatic System, Stamina, Urinary Tract, Glandular Disorder
✦ **Emotional Use:** Unconditional Love, Reduces Stress, Reduces Tension, Relaxation
✦ **Spiritual Use:** Mediation, Lucid Dreams, Earth Healing
✦ **Chakra:** Heart
✦ **Moh's Hardness:** 6-6.5
✦ **Zodiac:** Libra
✦ **Safe for Water:** Yes

GRAVE'S DISEASE (see hyperthyroidism)

-H-

<u>HAYFEVER (see allergies)</u>

HEART CONDITIONS

Other Crystals To Try: Rhodochrosite, Peridot, Green Aventurine, Rose Quartz

Rhodochrosite
- ✦ **Healing Use:** Heart Issues, Blood Pressure Regulator, Thyroid Balance, Memory, Lung, Respiratory Health, Prostate, Reproductive Organs, Ovarian Cancer, Veins, Migraine Relief, Infections, Kidney Disorder, Eye Infections, Cancer, Bladder Issues, Autoimmune Disorders, Asthma, Aging Process
- ✦ **Emotional Use:** Anxiety, Calming, Compassion, Creativity, Depression, Emotional Awareness, Emotional Balance, Fear, Forgiveness, Kindness, Letting Go, Love, Passion, Positivity, PTSD, Stress, Tension, Relationships, Self Acceptance, Self Worth, Self Confidence, Truth
- ✦ **Spiritual Use:** Divine Love, Dream Recall, Soulmate, Unconditional Love, Amplifying, Cleanses Aura, Balances Yin Energy, Cosmic Awareness
- ✦ **Chakra:** Heart
- ✦ **Moh's Hardness:** 3.5-4
- ✦ **Zodiac:** Leo/Scorpio
- ✦ **Safe for Water:** No

Peridot
- ✦ **Healing Use:** Heart Issues, Heart Burn, Indigestion, Balances Thyroid, Tissue Health, Lungs, Muscle Tone, Birthing Issues, Blood Sugar Regulation, Body, Breast Health, Detoxifying, Eye Disorders, Intestinal Disorders, Liver Issues, Smoking Addiction, Spleen, Trauma
- ✦ **Emotional Use:** Resentment, Stress, Diffuses Rage, Jealousy, Emotional Healing, Anger, Comforting, Coping with Grief, Eases Depression, Emotional Abuse, Emotional Healing, Irritability
- ✦ **Spiritual Use:** Visions, Abundance, Cleanses Aura, Creativity, Prosperity, Stimulates Spiritual Insight
- ✦ **Chakra:** Heart/Solar Plexus
- ✦ **Moh's Hardness:** 6.5-7
- ✦ **Zodiac:** Leo/Sagittarius/Scorpio/Virgo
- ✦ **Safe for Water:** No

HEADACHE

Other Crystals To Try: Smokey Quartz, Amethyst, Clear Quartz, Rose Quartz

Smokey Quartz
- ✦ **Healing Use:** Headaches, Knee, Leg, Hip, Abdomen, Dissolves Cramps, Grounding, Pain Reliever, Calmness, Strengthens back
- ✦ **Emotional Use:** Relieves Fear, Lifts Depression, Emotional Calmness, Absorbs Negativity and transmutes it to love
- ✦ **Spiritual Use:** Aura Protecting, Grounding, Healing the Earth, Enhances Dreams
- ✦ **Chakra:** Root
- ✦ **Moh's Hardness:** 7
- ✦ **Zodiac:** Scorpio/Sagittarius/Capricorn
- ✦ **Safe for Water:** Yes

HIVES/Urticaria (see allergies)

HYPERGLYCEMIA (HIGH BLOOD SUGAR)

Other Crystals To Try: Moss Agate, Pink Opal

HYPERTENSION (HIGH BLOOD PRESSURE

Other Crystals To Try: Blue Chalcedony, Bloodstone, Amethyst

HYPERTHYROIDISM (overactive)

Other Crystals To Try: Angelite, Blue Apatite, Aquamarine

Angelite
- ✦ **Healing Use:** Hyperthyroidism, Osteoporosis, Sleep, Throat, Water Retention
- ✦ **Emotional Use:** Truth, Acceptance, Compassion, Fear, Insecurity, Emotional Pain, Peace
- ✦ **Spiritual Use:** Telepathy, Visualization, Angel Communication, Astral Travel/Projection, Astrology, Attunement, Akashic Record, Connection to Spirit Guides, Connection to Totem Animals, Perception, Spiritual Protection
- ✦ **Chakra:** Throat/Crown
- ✦ **Moh's Hardness:** 3.5
- ✦ **Zodiac:** Aquarius
- ✦ **Safe for Water:** No

HYPOTHYROIDISM (underactive)

Other Crystals To Try: Lapis Lazuli, Blue Laced Agate, Chrysocolla

Lapis Lazuli

✦ **Healing Use:** Hypothyroidism, Pain, AIDS/HIVS, Asthma, Migraines, Brain Injury, Childbirth, Cramping, Dizziness, Ears, Epilepsy, Fainting, Headaches, Boosts Immune System, Insomnia, Menopause, Menstruation, Throat, Vertigo, Vomiting

✦ **Emotional Use:** Panic Attacks, Anxiety, Calm, Abuse, Depression, Emotional Healing, Grief, Hope, OCD, Stress, Self Confidence, Self Esteem, Suicidal Thoughts

✦ **Spiritual Use:** Appreciated, Communication w/Spirit, Etheric Balance, Intuition, Meditation, Protection, Psychic Protection, Spiritual Uplift, Stimulates Third Eye Chakra

✦ **Chakra:** Throat/Third Eye

✦ **Moh's Hardness:** 5-6

✦ **Zodiac:** Libra/Sagittarius

✦ **Safe for Water:** No

-I-

IMMUNE SYSTEM (boost)

Other Crystals To Try: Shungite, Bloodstone, Black Tourmaline

Shungite
- ✦ **Healing Use:** Detoxes Body, Boosts Immune System, Inflammation, Pain, Shields body from EMF, Purifies Water, Rids body of Virus/Bacteria, Asthma, Arthritis, Chronic Fatigue
- ✦ **Emotional Use:** Grounding, Protective, Removes Negativity
- ✦ **Spiritual Use:** Spiritual Evolution
- ✦ **Chakra:** Root
- ✦ **Moh's Hardness:** 3.5-4
- ✦ **Zodiac:** Cancer/Capricorn/Scorpio
- ✦ **Safe for Water:** Yes

IMPOTENCE (see erectile disfunction)

INDIGESTION

Other Crystals To Try: Blue Calcite, Citrine, Peridot

Blue Calcite
- ✦ **Healing Use:** Heart Burn, Indigestion, Acid Reflux, Aging Process, Cataracts, Eyes, Laryngitis, Lungs, Lower Blood Pressure, Addiction
- ✦ **Emotional Use:** Over-Active Mind, Anxiety, Calming, Encouragement, Emotional Pain, Stress, Relaxation, Clear Communication
- ✦ **Spiritual Use:** Clarity, Encouragement, Intuition, Insight
- ✦ **Chakra:** Throat/Third Eye
- ✦ **Moh's Hardness:** 2.5-3
- ✦ **Zodiac:** Cancer/Pisces
- ✦ **Safe for Water:** No

INSOMNIA

Other Crystals To Try: Howlite, Lepidolite, Amethyst, Moonstone

Howlite
- ✦ **Healing Use:** Relieves Insomnia, Relaxes Mind, Balances Calcium Levels, Bones, Teeth
- ✦ **Emotional Use:** Extremely Calming, Eliminates Rage
- ✦ **Spiritual Use:** Insight, Wisdom, Access Past Life, Spiritual Connection
- ✦ **Chakra:** Virgo/Gemini
- ✦ **Moh's Hardness:** 3.5
- ✦ **Zodiac:** Virgo/Gemini
- ✦ **Safe for Water:** No

IRON DEFICIENCY (see anemia)

IRRITABLE BOWL DISEASE (see Crohn's)

IRRITABLE BOWL SYNDROME (see Crohn's)

-K-

<u>KIDNEY STONES</u>

Other Crystals To Try: Garnet, Red Jasper, Hematite, Smokey Quartz

Garnet
- ✦ **Healing Use:** Kidney Stones, Stimulates Metabolism, Arthritis, Detoxing Blood, Sex Drive, Thyroid, Intestines, Colon, Hyperactivity, Anemia
- ✦ **Emotional Use:** Compassion, Honestly, Love, Self Confidence, Will Power, Courage, Hope
- ✦ **Spiritual Use:** Manifesting, Prosperity, Transformation, Unity, Protection
- ✦ **Chakra:** Root
- ✦ **Moh's Hardness:** 6- 7.5
- ✦ **Zodiac:** Aquarius/Capricorn/Leo/Virgo
- ✦ **Safe for Water:** No

-L-

<u>LARYNGITIS (see cough)</u>

<u>LIVER DISEASE</u>
Other Crystals To Try: Charoite, Malachite, Red Jasper, Tiger's Eye

Charoite
- ✦ **Healing Use:** Liver Issues, Pain, Arthritis, Autism, Blood Pressure Regulator, Headache, Migraines, High Blood Pressure, Insomnia, Mental Clarity, Gout, Kidneys
- ✦ **Emotional Use:** Creativity, Creative Expression, Release Negativity, Unconditional Love
- ✦ **Spiritual Use:** Clarity, Insight, Synchronicity, Truth
- ✦ **Chakra:** Third Eye/Crown
- ✦ **Moh's Hardness:** 5
- ✦ **Zodiac:** Sagittarius/Scorpio
- ✦ **Safe for Water:** No

LUNG DISEASE

Other Crystals To Try: Apophyllite, Vanadinite, Amber, Rose Quartz

Apophyllite
- ✦ **Healing Use:** Lungs, Addiction. Allergies, Asthma, Breathing Issues, Eye Issues, Fatigue, Foot Issues, Healing, Mental Clarity, Skin Infections
- ✦ **Emotional Use:** Anxiety, Release Negativity, Fear, Stress, Worry
- ✦ **Spiritual Use:** Akashic Records, Distance Healing, Meditation, Past Life Recall, Angel Communication, Clarity, Connection to Higher Self, Astral Projection/Travel, Introspection, Remote Viewing, Universal Love
- ✦ **Chakra:** Third Eye/Crown
- ✦ **Moh's Hardness:** 4.5-5
- ✦ **Zodiac:** Gemini/Libra
- ✦ **Safe for Water:** No

Vanadinite
- ✦ **Healing Use:** Lungs, Stabilizes Hormone Production, Aging, Menopause, EMF, Stimulates Mind, Helps you stay on Task, Energy Boost,
- ✦ **Emotional Use:** Creativity, Writers Block, Playfulness, Curiosity, Adventurous, Helps You Take Risks, Libido
- ✦ **Spiritual Use:** Connect with Inner Self, Grounding, Psychic Enhancement, Connect to Earth Energies
- ✦ **Chakra:** Root/Sacral
- ✦ **Moh's Hardness:** 3
- ✦ **Zodiac:** Virgo
- ✦ **Safe for Water:** No

LUPUS
Other Crystals To Try: Honey Calcite, Aquamarine, Bloodstone, Hematite

Honey Calcite
- ✦ **Healing Use:** Lupus, Blood Sugar Stabilizer, Exhaustion, Kidneys, Menopause, Ovaries, Cleanses Organs, Ulcers
- ✦ **Emotional Use:** Motivation, Dealing with Change, Energy, Will Power, Uplifting, Negativity
- ✦ **Spiritual Use:** Astral Projection, Balance, Consciousness, Enhances Meditation
- ✦ **Chakra:** Sacral/Solar Plexus
- ✦ **Moh's Hardness:** 2.5-3
- ✦ **Zodiac:** Cancer/Leo/Pisces
- ✦ **Safe for Water:** No

LYME DISEASE
Other Crystals To Try: Clear Quartz, Bloodstone

Clear Quartz
- ✦ **Healing Use:** Pain, Lyme, Burns, Heartburn, Boost Immune System, Memory, Sleep, Thyroid, Toothache, Vitality,
- ✦ **Emotional Use:** Acceptance, Balance, Friendship, Harmony, Joy, Stress, Stabilizing, Persevering
- ✦ **Spiritual Use:** Amplifies Wishes, Higher Self, Humility, Connection to Spirit Guides, Telepathy, Unity, Awareness
- ✦ **Chakra:** All/Crown
- ✦ **Moh's Hardness:** 7
- ✦ **Zodiac:** All Signs
- ✦ **Safe for Water:** Yes

-M-

MENIERE'S DISEASE
Other Crystals To Try: Dioptase, Rose Quartz, Snowflake Obsidian, Lapis Lazuli, Rhodonite

Dioptase
- ✦ **Healing Use:** Meniere's, Pain Relief, Muscle Issues, Lungs, PMS, Headache, Migraine, Blood Pressure Regulator, Cancer, Healing Wounds, Heart Issues, Wounds, AIDS/HIV, Detoxifying, Emphysema, Heart Burn, Liver Issues, Tumor
- ✦ **Emotional Use:** Compassion, Emotional Balance, Joy, Reduces Stress, Depression
- ✦ **Spiritual Use:** Cleansing Aura
- ✦ **Chakra:** Heart
- ✦ **Moh's Hardness:** 5
- ✦ **Zodiac:** Sagittarius/Scorpio
- ✦ **Safe for Water:** No

<u>MENOPAUSE</u>

Other Crystals To Try: Moonstone, Citrine, Garnet, Rose Quartz, Lepidolite

Moonstone
- ✦ **Healing Use:** Menstrual Cramps, Menopause, Indigestion, Upper Digestive Tract, Reproductive System, Pregnancy, Child Birth, Lactation, PMS, Insomnia, Obesity, Stomach, Sting/Bites, MS, Infertility
- ✦ **Emotional Use:** Stabilizes Emotions, Release Tension, Empathy, Stress, Centering, Fear of Dark, Hope, Inspiration, Postpartum Depression
- ✦ **Spiritual Use:** Harness Power of The Moon, Intuition, Imagination, Lucid Dreaming, Enhances Psychic , Clairvoyance, Energy Work, Increases Awareness, Psychic Protection
- ✦ **Chakra:** Crown/Sacral
- ✦ **Moh's Hardness:** 6-6.5
- ✦ **Zodiac:** Cancer/Leo/Scorpio
- ✦ **Safe for Water:** No

MENSTRUAL CRAMPS

Other Crystals To Try: Selenite, Moonstone, Chrysocolla, Carnelian

Selenite

✦ **Healing Use:** PMS, Back Issues, Bone Disorders, Bone Strengthening, Cancer, Epilepsy, Healing, Infection, Insomnia, Muscular Issues, Psoriasis, Sleep, Spinal Strengthening, Spine Health, Tumor, Ulcers

✦ **Emotional Use:** Self Worth, Chaos, Forgiveness, Harmony, Honestly, Positive Energy, Stress, Self Confidence

✦ **Spiritual Use:** Connection to Angels, Cleanses Aura, Communication w/Higher Self, Connection with Higher Realms, Increases Intuition, Meditation, Past Life Recall, Raises Vibration, Reiki, Release Negativity, Shifts Consciousness, White Light Energy

✦ **Chakra:** Crown/Third Eye

✦ **Moh's Hardness:** 2

✦ **Zodiac:** Taurus

✦ **Safe for Water:** No

MIGRAINE

Other Crystals To Try: Topaz, Rose Quartz, Lapis Lazuli, Amethyst, Fluorite

Topaz
- ✦ **Healing Use:** Migraine, Headache, Concentration, Detoxifying, Digestion, Eating Disorders, Glandular Disorders, Gout, Increases Metabolism, Night Terrors, Ovarian Cysts, Pancreases, Heals Tissue
- ✦ **Emotional Use:** Courage, Fear, Fear of Dark
- ✦ **Spiritual Use:** Abundance, Clairvoyance, Manifestions
- ✦ **Chakra:** Crown/Sacral/Solar Plexus
- ✦ **Moh's Hardness:** 8
- ✦ **Zodiac:** Sagittarius
- ✦ **Safe for Water:** No

MULTIPLE SCLEROSIS (MS)

Other Crystals To Try: Black Tourmaline, Carnelian, Red Jasper, Lapis Lazuli

Black Tourmaline
- ✦ **Healing Use:** MS, Motion Sickness, Torn Muscle, Muscle Strain, Arthritis, Dyslexia, Aids IBS, Protection from EMF
- ✦ **Emotional Use:** Releases Tension, Balances Yin/Yang, OCD
- ✦ **Spiritual Use:** Protective, Grounding, Psychic Attack, Absorbs Negativity
- ✦ **Chakra:** Root
- ✦ **Moh's Hardness:** 7
- ✦ **Zodiac:** Capricorn
- ✦ **Safe for Water:** No

-P-

PAIN

Other Crystals To Try: Boji Stones, Smokey Quartz, Clear Quartz, Amber, Fluorite, Hematite

Boji Stones/Moqui Marbles
- ✦ **Healing Use:** Pain Relief, Insomnia
- ✦ **Emotional Use:** Relationship Help, Centering, Balances Yin/Yang Energies, Eases Mind
- ✦ **Spiritual Use:** Protection, Grounding, Balances Chakras
- ✦ **Chakra:** Root
- ✦ **Moh's Hardness:** 4-5
- ✦ **Zodiac:** Aquarius/Aries/Capricorn/Libra
- ✦ **Safe for Water:** No

PNEUMONIA (see cough)

POST TRAUMATIC STRESS DISORDER (PTSD) (see pain/anxiety)

<u>POSTNATAL DEPRESSION (see anxiety)</u>

<u>PROSTATE (see frequent urination)</u>

<u>PSORIASIS (see eczema)</u>

-R-

<u>RHEUMATOID ARTHRITIS (see Arthritis)</u>

-S-

<u>SHINGLES</u>
Other Crystals To Try: Jade, Blue Laced Agate, Chrysoprase, Rose Quartz

Jade
- ✦ **Healing Use:** Shingles, Skin Infections, Blood Pressure, Bone Disorders, Cellular Disorders, Cramps, Reproductive Organs.
- ✦ **Emotional Use:** Relationships, Love, Harmony, Abundance, Prosperity
- ✦ **Spiritual Use:** Lucid Dreaming
- ✦ **Chakra:** Heart/Root
- ✦ **Moh's Hardness:** 6.5-7
- ✦ **Zodiac:** Aries
- ✦ **Safe for Water:** No

<u>SIBO</u> (see Crohn's)

SINUSITIS
Other Crystals To Try: Emerald, Amethyst, Labradorite

Emerald
✦ **Healing Use:** Sinus Issues, Colds, Flu, Cancer, Arthritis, Blood Pressure Regulator, Emphysema, Eye Disorders, Fever, Heart Issues, Boosts Immune System, Liver Disorders, Improves Memory, Nausea, Toxins, Vomiting, Weakness
✦ **Emotional Use:** Tranquility, Inspiration, Honesty, Calming, Guilt, Coping with Grief, Compassion, Abundance, Prosperity
✦ **Spiritual Use:** Visons , Karma, Serenity, Clarity, Clairvoyance
✦ **Chakra:** Heart
✦ **Moh's Hardness:** 7.5-8
✦ **Zodiac:** Aries/Gemini/Taurus
✦ **Safe for Water:** No

SORE THROAT (see cough)

STOMACHACHE/ABDOMINAL PAIN

Other Crystals To Try: Turritella Agate, Citrine, Amber, Carnelian, Chrysoprase

Turritella Agate
- ✦ **Healing Use:** Stomach issues, Digestion, Pain in Stomach, Gastroenteritis, Fatigue, Absorption of Vitamins, Swelling in Hands/Feet, Gallstones, Skin Rash, Insect Bite, Varicose Veins, Sexual Disfunction, Strengthens Heart, Fever, Epilepsy, Sleepwalking, Safe Travels, Fertility
- ✦ **Emotional Use:** Healing Past, Stability, Maturity, Fears, Negativity, Balance
- ✦ **Spiritual Use:** Awareness, Inner Stability, Spiritual Growth, Past Lives, Communication w/Mineral & Plant Kingdom
- ✦ **Chakra:** Root
- ✦ **Moh's Hardness:** 7
- ✦ **Zodiac:** Gemini
- ✦ **Safe for Water:** Yes

STRESS (see anxiety)

<u>STROKE</u>

Other Crystals To Try: Chiastolite, Lapis Lazuli, Garnet

Chiastolite
✦ **Healing Use:** Stroke, Paralysis, Nerve Damage, Muscle Weakness, Muscle Spams, Gout, Rheumatoid Diseases, Increases Vibrational Field After Being ill, Regulates Nervous System & Energetic Field
✦ **Emotional Use:** Protection, Psychic Attack, Strength, Wards off Curses, Grounding, Earth Connection, Depression, Fear
✦ **Spiritual Use:** Connection to Elements, Cleanses Aura, Clears Blockages in Chakras & Meridians, Protects Against Energy Drain, Activates Higher Chakras, Connection with Spiritual Realm, Attracts Light, Akashic Records
✦ **Chakra:** Root
✦ **Moh's Hardness:** 7.5
✦ **Zodiac:** Virgo
✦ **Safe for Water:** No

-T-

THYROID (see hyper/hypothyroidism)

TUBERCULOSIS (TB)
Other Crystals To Try: Morganite, Amber, Emerald, Dioptase, Topaz

Morganite
- ✦ **Healing Use:** TB, Throat, Lungs, Impotence, Heart, Abdominal Pain, Asthma, Dying Process, Emphysema, Muscular, Skeletal, Sexual Abuse
- ✦ **Emotional Use:** Coping with Changes, Depression, Emotional Release, Forgiveness, Love, Motivation, Stress, Releasing Toxic Patterns, Self Acceptance, Self Love, Unconditional Love
- ✦ **Spiritual Use:** Soul Retrieval, Angel Communication, Connection with Higher Source, Divine Love, Connection with Spirit
- ✦ **Chakra:** Heart
- ✦ **Moh's Hardness:** 7.5-8
- ✦ **Zodiac:** Libra
- ✦ **Safe for Water:** No

TUMOR

Other Crystals To Try: Sunstone, Hematite, Amethyst, Fluorite

Sunstone
- ✦ **Healing Use:** Tumor, Digestion, Kidneys, Liver, Stomach, Tension, Ulcers, Throat, Sexual Issues, Aches, Pain
- ✦ **Emotional Use:** Joy, Happiness, Harmony, Empowerment, Encouragement, Abundance, Leadership
- ✦ **Spiritual Use:** Aura Cleanser, Right use of Will, Good Luck
- ✦ **Chakra:** Sacral
- ✦ **Moh's Hardness:** 6-6.5
- ✦ **Zodiac:** Leo/Libra
- ✦ **Safe for Water:** No

-U-

ULCERTATIVE COLITIS (see Crohn's)

URINARY TRACT INFECTION (UTI)
Other Crystals To Try: Amber, Carnelian

-V-

VERTIGO
Other Crystals To Try: Rose Quartz, Lapis Lazuli, Malachite

Rose Quartz
- ✦ **Healing Use:** Vertigo, Burns, Bulimia, Cough, Skin, Alzheimer's, PTSD, Shingles, Emphysema, Heart, Lungs, Fertility, Soothes Complexion
- ✦ **Emotional Use:** Unconditional Love, Relaxing, Emotional Balance, Self Care, Acceptance, Selflessness
- ✦ **Spiritual Use:** Divine Love, Increases Positive Energy, Spiritual Love, Peace, Inner Healing
- ✦ **Chakra:** Heart
- ✦ **Moh's Hardness:** 7
- ✦ **Zodiac:** Libra/Taurus
- ✦ **Safe for Water:** Yes

VIRUS (see cold)

-W-

WEIGHT LOSS

Other Crystals To Try: Yellow Apatite, Unakite, Prehnite

Yellow Apatite

- ✦ **Healing Use:** Appetite Suppressant, Broken Bones, Arthritis, Muscle, Tissue, Liver, Pancreas, Spleen, Teeth
- ✦ **Emotional Use:** Positivity, Apathy, Depression, Emotional Blockages, Motivation
- ✦ **Spiritual Use:** Psychic Abilities, Past Life Recall, Allow you to Let Go
- ✦ **Chakra:** Solar Plexus
- ✦ **Moh's Hardness:** 5
- ✦ **Zodiac:** Gemini
- ✦ **Safe for Water:** No

Unakite

- ✦ **Healing Use:** Enhances Metabolism, Addiction, Alcoholism, Colds, Flu, Heart, Infertility, Aids in Healthy Pregnancy, Menstration, Reproductive Organs, Skin Infections, Tissues Healing, Healing
- ✦ **Emotional Use:** Emotional Healing, Motivation, Connection to Earth Energies
- ✦ **Spiritual Use:** Actives Will, Increases Intuition, Meditation, Past Life Recall, Rebirth
- ✦ **Chakra:** Heart
- ✦ **Moh's Hardness:** 6-7
- ✦ **Zodiac:** Scorpio
- ✦ **Safe for Water:** No

<u>WHOOPING COUGH (see cough)</u>

Ailments List-Crystals

- **ADHD:** Amethyst, Lepidolite, Hematite, Amazonite, Rose Quartz
- **Allergies:** Moss Agate, Carnelian, Red Jasper, Petrified Wood, Turquoise
- **Alzheimer's :** Rose Quartz, Lepidolite, Rhodonite, Rutilated Quartz, Amber
- **Anemia:** Bloodstone, Hematite, Tiger's Eye, Garnet, Copper
- **Anxiety:** Lepidolite, Amethyst, Blue Laced Agate, Chyroprase, Sunstone
- **Arthritis:** Fluorite, Azurite, Malachite, Rhodonite, Copper
- **Asthma:** Amber, Rose Quartz, Tiger's Eye, Jade
- **Autism:** Blue Apatite, Tigers Eye, Red Jasper, Jade, Charoite
- **Bacteria Infection:** Green Calcite, Clear Quartz, Amber, Nephrite Jade
- **Bipolar disorder:** Lepidolite, Snowflake Obsidian, Charoite, Kunzite
- **Blood Pressure** (see hypertension)
- **Boost Memory:** (see Alzheminers)
- **Brusing:** Hematite, Angelite, Fluorite
- **Bursitis:** Copper, Clear Quartz
- **Cancer:** Citrine, Amethyst, Smokey Quartz, Emerald, Carnelian
- **Cholesterol (high) :** Green Aventurine, Fluorite
- **Constipation:** Citrine, Amber, Ruby, Red Jasper
- **Common Cold:** Carnelian, Moss Agate, Ametrine, Emerald
- **Cough:** Aquamarine, Blue Laced Agate, Amber, Rose Quartz
- **Crohn's disease:** Chrysocolla, Hawk's Eye (Blue Tiger's Eye), Yellow Jasper, Peridot, Green Aventurine, Blue Chalcedony
- **Dementia:** (see Alzheimers)
- **Depression**: (see Anxiety)
- **Diabetes:** Citrine, Emerald, Pink Opal, Jade, Clear Quartz
- **Eczema :** Amethyst, Green Aventurine, Fluorite
- **Erectile disfunction:** Variscite, Carnelian, Sunstone, Rose Quartz

- **Epilepsy:** Red Jasper, Hematite, Amethyst, Black Tourmaline, Lapis Lazuli
- **Fever:** Blue Chalcedony, Hematite, Carnelian, Aquamarine, Pietersite
- **Fibromyalgia:** Selenite, Rutilated Quartz, Amethyst, Malachite, Emerald, Hematite, Black Tourmaline, Clear Quartz
- **Flu** (see common cold)
- **Frequent Urination (at night):** Black Obsidian, Dragon's Eye (Red Tiger's Eye)
- **Gallbladder (Gallstones) :** Canelian, Danburite, Jade, Citrine
- **Gout:** Bornite, Chaistolite, Prehnite, Labrodorite, Chysoprase
- **Graves' disease: (See Hyperthyroidism)**
- **Hay fever (see allergies)**
- **Heart conditions:** Green Aventurine, Rhodochrosite, Peridot, Rose Quartz
- **Headache:** Amethyst, Smokey Quartz, Clear Quartz, Rose Quartz
- **Hives/Urticaria: (see Allergies)**
- **Hyperglycemia (high blood sugar):** Moss Agate, Pink Opal, Chrysocolla
- **Hypertension (high blood pressure):** Blue Chalcedony, Bloodstone, Amethyst, Chrysocolla
- **Hyperthyroidism (Over active thyroid) :** Aquamarine, Angelite, Blue Apatite
- **Hypothyroidism (under active thyroid):** Blue Laced Agate, Lapis Lazuli, Chrysocolla
- **Immune System (boost):** Bloodstone, Shungite, Black Tourmaline
- **Impotence** (see Erectile disfunction)
- **Indigestion (Heart Burn):** Blue Calcite, Citrine, Peridot
- **Insomnia:** Howlite, Lepidolite, Amethyst, Moonstone, Selenite
- **Iron deficiency** (see anemia)
- **Irritable Bowl Disease (IBD)** (see Crohn's)
- **Irritable Bowel Syndrome (IBS)** (see Crohn's)
- **Kidney stones:** (see Gallbladder)
- **Laryngitis :** (see cough)
- **Liver disease:** Charoite, Malachite, Red Jasper, Tiger's Eye, Emerald

- o **Lung disease:** Apophylllite, Vanadinite, Amber, Rose Quartz
- o **Lupus:** Honey Calcite, Aquamarine, Bloodstone, Hematite
- o **Lyme disease :** Bloodstone, Clear Quartz
- o **Meniere's Disease :** Dioptase, Rose Quartz, Snowflake Obsidian, Lapis Lazuli, Rhodonite
- o **Menopause:** Citrine, Garnet, Moonstone, Rose Quartz, Lepidolite
- o **Menstrual cramps:** Moonstone, Chrysocolla, Carnelian, Selenite, Ruby
- o **Migraine:** Lapis Lazuli, Topaz, Rose Quartz, Amethyst, Fluorite
- o **Multiple sclerosis (MS) :** Carnelian, Black Tourmaline, Red Jasper, Lapis Lazuli, Jade, Hematite
- o **Pain:** Clear Quartz, Smokey Quartz, Amber, Flourite, Hematite, Boji Stones, Howlite
- o **Pneumonia: (also see cough)**
- o **Post traumatic stress disorder (PTSD)** (See Anxiety)
- o **Postnatal depression:** (see anxiety)
- o **Prostate:** (see frequent urination)
- o **Psoriasis** (see eczema)
- o **Rheumatoid arthritis** (see arthritis)
- o **Seasickness:** Aquamarine
- o **Shingles:** Blue Laced Agate, Chrysoprase, Jade, Rose Quartz
- o **SIBO** (See Crohn's)
- o **Sinusitis:** Fluorite, Emerald, Amethyst, Labradorite, Jade
- o **Sore throat** (see cough)
- o **Stomachache/Abdominal pain:** Citrine, Amber, Carnelian, Turritella Agate
- o **Stress:** (see Anxiety)
- o **Stroke:** Chaistolite, Lapis Lazuli, Garnet
- o **Thyroid (see hyper/hypo-thyroidism)**
- o **Tuberculosis (TB):** Amber, Morganite, Emerald, Dioptase, Topaz
- o **Tumors:** Hematite, Bloodstone, Malachite, Sunstone, Fluorite, Amethyst
- o **Ulcerative Colitis (see Crohn's)**
- o **Urinary tract infection (UTI) :** Amber, Clear Quartz, Carnelian
- o **Vertigo:** Lapis Lazuli, Rose Quartz, Malachite (see Menieres Disease)
- o **Virus** (see cold)

- o **Weight loss:** Yellow Apatite, Unakite, Prehnite, Iolite
- o **Whooping cough:** (See Cough)

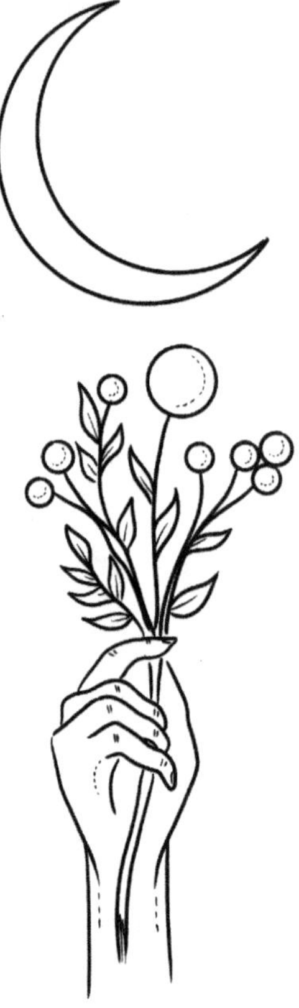

CONCLUSION

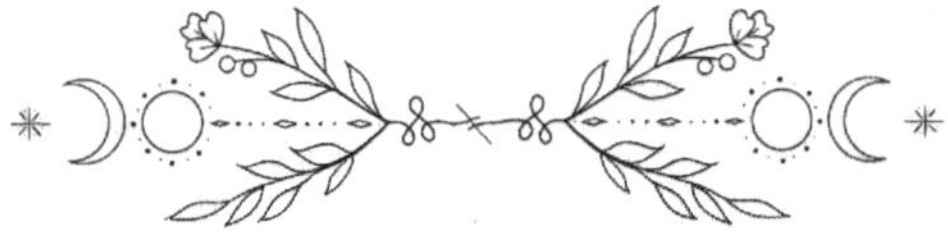

I hope you found lots of useful information in this book to help you heal yourself holistically!

Always believe in your magick, and the power of Plants and Minerals! It's truly amazing the world we get to inhabit! We are never alone in our healing process!!

Gaia has supplied us with an abundance of ways to heal ourselves! It's all about tapping into the source within us, listening, and following the advice our Soul provides.

Healing yourself naturally is so rewarding… and you will live a happier, healthier life because of it!

My wish is that you embrace this knowledge and give thanks for all the amazing ways we have been provided for!

Wishing you and your family a life time full of health, happiness and of course… magick!

ACKNOWLEDGMENT

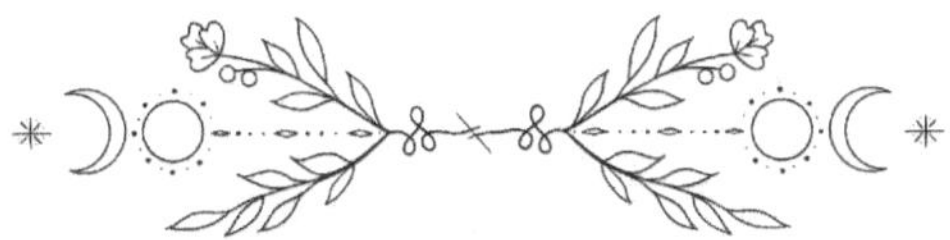

A special Thank you to My Hubby Jared and Daughter Kelsey for not only supporting all my MANY adventures…but for your contribution on both of my books!

Jared… thank you for sharing your artistic talents on the Cover of the book and the lovely artwork throughout!

Kelsey… thanks so much for sharing your talents by doing all the beautiful photography in the book!

You are both the best and I love you so much!! I appreciate you both more than you'll ever know!!

Thanks for playing a loving supportive role in my life!
Love you both to the Moon & Back again!!

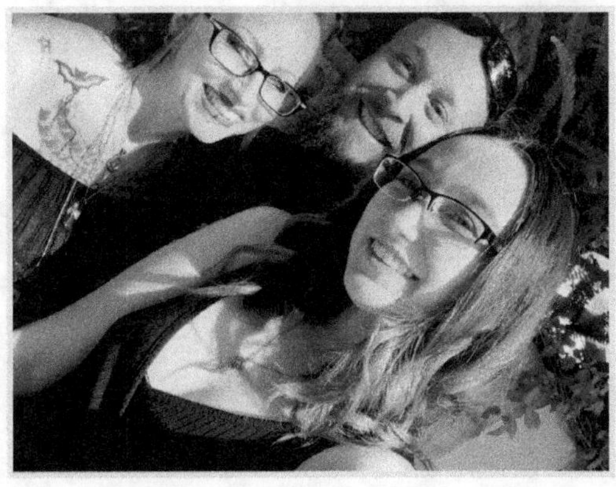

THE AUTHOR

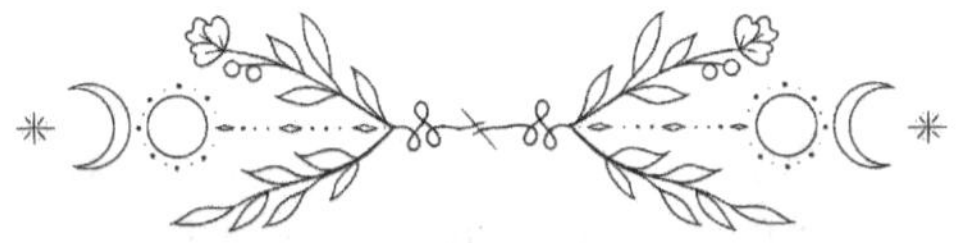

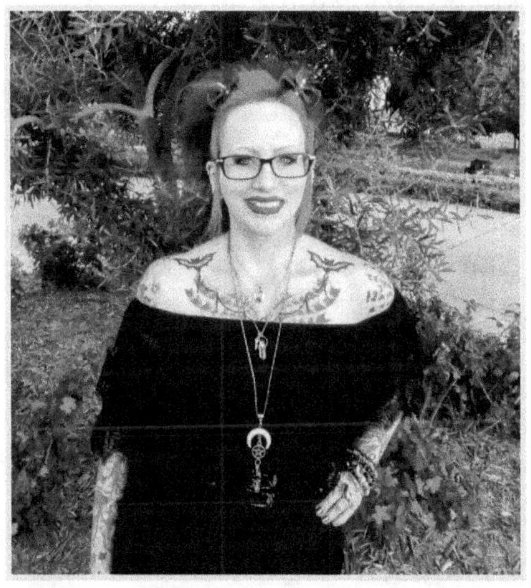

B ridget M. Shoup is known as "The Crystal Healing Gypsy".

She is a Wife, Mommy, Minister, Crystal Reiki Master, and Solitary Eclectic Witch, residing in California.

She has always had a passion to help others! Her life's mission is to reach out and assist as many people as she can life a happier, healthier, holistic lifestyle. One ways she does this is by teaching others at the many events she hosts, sharing her knowledge and sound healing.

Bridget had the beginning of her spiritual awakening in 2013. By 2016, she was full fledged into learning every aspect she could about Crystals and their healing powers!

From there it lead her to rediscovering plant medicine and working in all realms within the Metaphysical arena.

She has been certified in a vast variety of metaphysical offerings. Services ranging from Crystal Healing, Sound Healing, Tarot & Numerology Readings, NLP, Aromatherapy, Herbology, Moon Mystic, and Life Coach. She is certified in all of these subjects and enjoys helping others on their journey.
She also is a Crystal Reiki Master, Certified Metaphysical Practitioner as well as an Ordained Minister.

As she continued on her life's path, she had witness first hand the healing powers of Crystals and knew she needed to share it with the world!
With this strong desire to serve others… in 2016 her company, B*MoonStruck was born (www.BMoonStruck.com).

Being deeply connected to her Spirit Guides, she was prompted in 2019 to write her first book called "Crystal Clear Enlightenment" a Guide to Spiritual Growth!
This book is her way of helping others along their path, as it can be a confusing time.

Again inspiration strikes in 2020 to write her second book, to again assist others. This time incorporating Herbs and Crystals together in an effort to share her knowledge on how to heal holistically!

Helping others enjoy their life time is a goal for Bridget.
But she also makes sure she has time for herself, to hone her practice.
Some of the things she enjoys are meditation, yoga, Qigong, art, music, hiking, spell work, writing, working with Crystals, gardening, harvesting Herbs, and sending as much time as she can with her family!

When she isn't doing that, she is thrilled to serve others with healing sessions through her company, B*MoonStruck.
(www.BMoonStruck.com)

She also runs an Etsy shop called "Bridget's Brew", where she offers potions (essential oil blends w/Crystal's infused) and other magickal items!
(www.etsy.com/shop/BridgetsBrew)

On the weekends you can usually find Bridget Officiating Weddings!! This is so much fun for her, as she loves to see people in love! She does this through her company called "Magickal Weddings". (https://magickalweddings.wixsite.com/bybridget)

Bridget is so happy to finally understand her Soul's desire! She is so excited to be able to share with you her journey, in hopes to help you on yours!

CHECK OUT MY OTHER BOOK

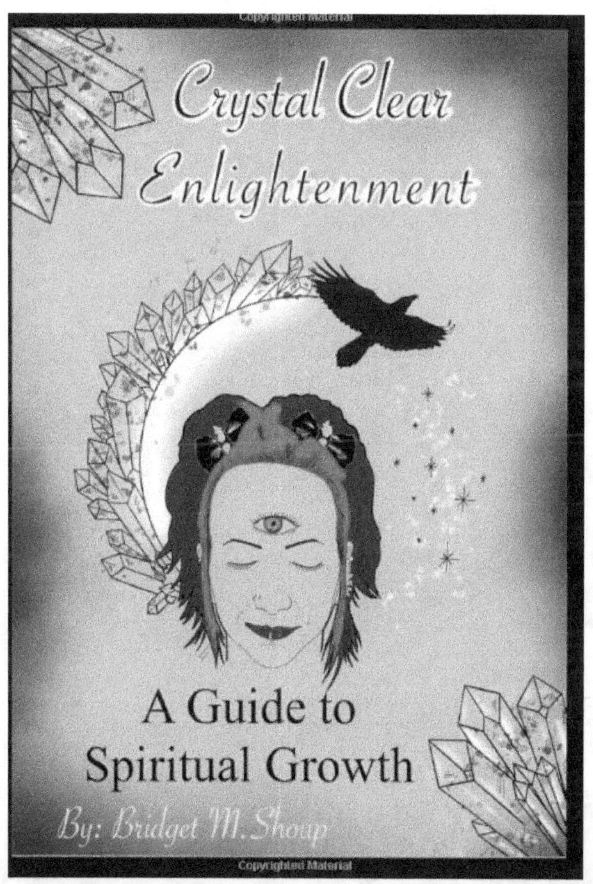

"Crystal Clear Enlightenment"
A Guide to Spiritual Growth

Order Online @Amazon.com

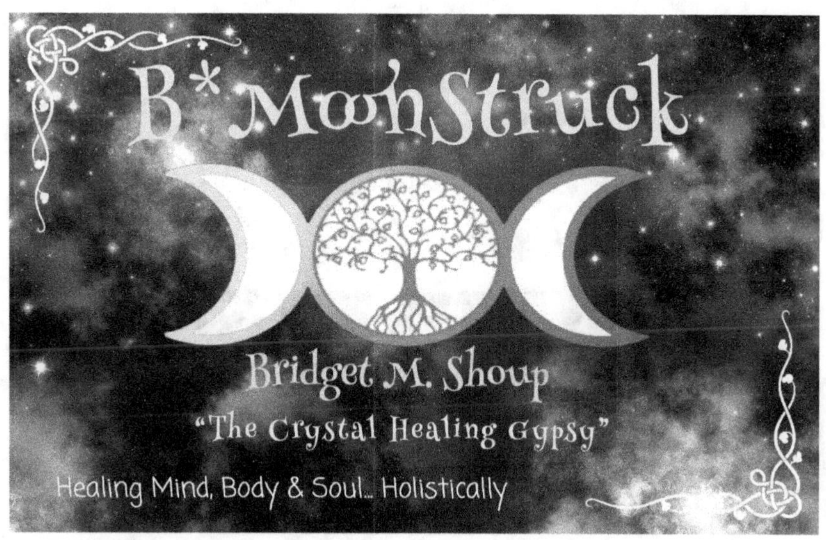

VISIT MY SITE:

www.BMoonStruck.com

INDEX

AILMENT INDEX

HERBAL INDEX

- Mugwort: 108
- Noni: 111
- Oregano oil: 87
- Panax Ginseng: 80
- Poria cocos: 80
- Poppy Seed: 111
- Psyllium Husk: 86, 96, 104
- Qing Dai: 20, 89
- Reishi Mushroom: 84
- Rhodiola Rosea: 74, 82, 116
- Rosemary: 61, 75, 76
- Saffron: 119
- Sage: 59, 137-138
- Saw Palmetto: 94
- Schisandra chinensis: 80
- Selenium: 100
- Skullcap: 78-79, 84, 89, 92, 96, 103
- Slippery Elm: 19-20, 86, 88-89
- Soursop: 84
- Star Anise: 62
- St. John's Wort: 82, 112
- Stinging Nettel: 75, 79
- Thyme: 84-85
- Triphala: 86
- Turmeric: 19-20, 47, 75, 79, 83-85, 89, 93, 95-96, 106, 110, 111, 119
- Valerian Root: 103
- Vitamin B-Complex: 74, 78
- Vitamin B6: 74, 79
- Vitamin B12: 20, 84, 89, 113
- Vitamin C: 20, 88, 95
- Vitamin D: 20, 80, 87
- Vitamin D3: 84, 89, 91, 93
- Vitamin E: 91
- Willow Bark: 111
- Witch Hazel: 91
- Wormwood: 19-20, 89
- Zinc: 87-88, 101, 113

CRYSTAL INDEX